"Martina's low-carb creations taste as spectacular as they look. She's dedicated to providing accurate, reliable information to people interested in following a healthy, carbohydrate-restricted lifestyle."
—Franziska Spritzler, R.D., C.D.E., author of *The Low Carb Dietitian's Guide to Health and Beauty*

"You're in good hands with Martina Slajerova and *The KetoDiet Cookbook*. Not only are her recipes reliable and true to the keto way of life, but they are mouthwateringly delicious. Lifestyle change is hard, but Martina makes it so much easier."
—Carolyn Ketchum, founder of AllDayIDreamAboutFood.com

"Low-carb diets are an invaluable tool in dealing with health conditions such as obesity, diabetes, metabolic syndrome, lipid disorders, epilepsy, and increasingly, cancer. Martina's work, including her blog, book, and apps, has been a real gem for the low-carb community. Her real-food approach and attention to detail sets her work apart from many others."
—Eugene J. Fine, M.D., professor of radiology at Albert Einstein College of Medicine

"Just like Martina's blog and app, her new cookbook is an amazing resource for anyone interested in healthy living, with easy to follow recipes and beautiful photography."
—Alex Pearlman, Ph.D., cancer biologist at Albert Einstein College of Medicine

"Martina's popular KetoDiet blog has been a wonderful resource for those following a healthy Paleo/primal, low-carb diet. She provides a wealth of information for successfully implementing a ketogenic diet and her recipes have become staples for those seeking low-carb alternatives for their favorite foods. This cookbook is a must for any low-carb cook's collection."
—Lisa MarcAurele, founder of LowCarbYum.com

"Martina's newest cookbook is not just a comprehensive guide to eating for the ketogenic diet, it is also gorgeous eye candy! It is sheer pleasure to browse through her gorgeous photographs while drooling over the delicious recipes. I love Martina's recipes especially because they are made with wholesome, real food ingredients. Every recipe is explained clearly and well organized, so you can always get great results when making them at home. If you are following a keto or low-carb lifestyle, this book is a must have!"
—Vivica Menegaz, founder of TheNourishedCaveman.com

"With its amazing quality, this book simply stands out from the gray crowd of the numerous low-carb and ketogenic cookbooks. That's why I am happy to recommend the book to anybody who seeks the latest information about healthy nutrition and the best, carefully developed ketogenic recipes."
—Elviira Krebber, founder of LowCarbSoSimple.com

I dedicate this book to Nikos, my fiancé
and best friend. Without your patience
and enless support, I would have never
chased my dreams to have a job I love.

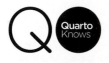

Quarto is the authority on a wide range of topics.

Quarto educates, entertains and enriches the lives of
our readers—enthusiasts and lovers of hands-on living.

www.QuartoKnows.com

© 2016 Quarto Publishing Group USA Inc.
Text © 2016 Martina Slajerova
Photography © 2016 Quarto Publishing Group USA Inc.

First published in the United States of America in 2016 by
Fair Winds Press, an imprint of
Quarto Publishing Group USA Inc.
100 Cummings Center
Suite 406-L
Beverly, Massachusetts 01915-6101
Telephone: (978) 282-9590
Fax: (978) 283-2742
www.QuartoKnows.com
Visit our blogs at www.QuartoKnows.com

19 18 17 16   2 3 4 5

ISBN: 978-1-59233-701-9

Digital edition published in 2016
eISBN: 978-1-62788-790-8

Library of Congress Cataloging-in-Publication Data
Slajerova, Martina.
  The keto diet cookbook : 150 grain-free, sugar-free, and starch-free
recipes for your low-carb, paleo, or ketogenic lifestyle / Martina
Slajerova.
      pages cm
  ISBN 978-1-59233-701-9
  1. Reducing diets. 2. Ketogenic diet. 3. Low-carbohydrate diet. I.
Title.
  RM222.2.S574 2015
  641.5'6383--dc23

                                    2015024238

Cover and Book design by Emily Portnoi
Photography by Martina Slajerova

Printed and bound in China

Disclaimer

*The resources listed in this book are not intended to be fully
systematic or complete, nor does inclusion here imply any
endorsement or recommendation. We make no warranties, express
or implied, about the value or utility for any purpose of the
information and resources contained herein. It is recommended you
first consult with your doctor about this diet plan, especially if you
are pregnant or nursing or have any health issues such as diabetes,
thyroid dysfunction, etc., as your health care provider may need to
adjust the medication you are taking. Further, this book is not
intended for the treatment or prevention of any disease, nor as a
substitute for medical treatment, nor as an alternative to medical
advice. Recommendations outlined herein should not be adopted
without a full review of the scientific references given and
consultation with a health care professional.*

The KetoDiet Cookbook

MORE THAN 150 DELICIOUS LOW-CARB, HIGH-FAT RECIPES
for Maximum Weight Loss *and* Improved Health

MARTINA
SLAJEROVA

FAIR WINDS

CONTENTS

INTRODUCTION

INTRODUCTION

I've always been passionate about cooking, health, and nutrition: in fact, I've been collecting recipes and articles since I was a teenager. When I was younger, like lots of girls my age, I followed what I perceived to be a balanced diet to manage my weight and stay healthy. I watched my calorie intake and chose low-fat and whole-grain products. I avoided foods high in saturated fats and cholesterol, and I exercised up to six times a week to keep extra pounds off. Like so many other people, I was convinced that eating less and exercising more was the best approach to staying healthy and slim.

Then, in 2011, I started having fatigue issues, and I frequently felt unwell. Although I still watched what I ate and exercised regularly, my weight began to climb. After several tests, I was finally diagnosed with Hashimoto's hypothyroidism. I felt terrible. I couldn't understand what I had done wrong: I was eating healthy foods, and I was exercising almost every day—yet I got sick. I knew that Hashimoto's, as well as other autoimmune disorders, could be triggered by lifestyle and diet factors—but that didn't make any sense to me, either, since I thought I had done everything I possibly could to stay healthy. So, I became determined to find out how to actively improve my condition rather than just relying on medication to manage it.

I soon realized that I wouldn't be able to maintain a healthy weight unless I changed my eating habits. From the day of my diagnosis, I researched different diets and food philosophies to try to figure out what might work best for me. After some trial and error, I discovered low-carb eating. At first, I was skeptical about this approach. All I'd heard about low-carb diets up to that point was that they were an unhealthy fad. But after months of reading books and medical articles, I realized I was wrong. Low-carb eating isn't just a diet; it's a lifestyle approach that can offer great health benefits. Calorie-counting is a thing of the past, my energy levels are back to normal, and I don't exercise more than three times a week. And I've never felt better.

Following a low-carb, paleo/primal diet plan helps me maintain a healthy weight while eating real food, and it inspires the dishes I create. My recipes are all grain-free, sugar-free, and gluten-free, and many of them include a dairy-free alternative. I always opt for grass-fed beef and butter; raw, hormone-free dairy; and healthy fats like coconut oil.

This book will walk you through the guidelines and benefits of the ketogenic diet, and it'll show you how to make more than 150 delicious low-carb recipes for everything from breakfast to dessert—plus some low-carb staples that are easy to make at home.

Simply put, low-carb eating has changed my life. I hope *The KetoDiet Cookbook* will do the same for you!

Martina Slajerova

Chapter One:

WHAT IS THE KETOGENIC DIET?

For decades, we've been given the wrong advice: Eat less, avoid dietary fats, and exercise more. Today, carbohydrates constitute the majority of our diet, and that has significant implications for hormone balance. Insulin, which is also responsible for storing fat in our bodies, is greatly affected by excessive carbohydrate consumption. And that means that carbohydrates are, without doubt, the most fattening element in our diets.

Yet, the standard dietary guidelines most of us are familiar with advise that we follow a high-carb, moderate-protein, and low-fat diet (45% to 65% calories from carbohydrates, 10% to 35% calories from protein, and 20% to 35% calories from fat). Contrary to these macronutrient recommendations, the ketogenic diet is high in fat, moderate in protein, and low in carbs. The macronutrient ratio in terms of calories typically sits within the following ranges:

60% to 75% (or even more) of calories from fat

15% to 30% of calories from protein

5% to 10% of calories from carbs

With this macronutrient intake, the ketogenic diet achieves weight loss and health benefits by inducing a metabolic state known as ketosis, which is usually achieved at a level of about 50 grams of total carbohydrates a day (20 to 30 grams of net carbohydrates). Ketosis causes the liver to produce ketone bodies—molecules created by the body for energy during periods of fasting or carbohydrate restriction—which shifts the body's metabolism away from glucose (the primary energy source derived from carbs) and toward burning fat.

One significant health benefit of the ketogenic diet is that it enhances the individual's ability to build and preserve muscle tissue. And it's not only an effective weight-loss tool; it's also been shown to improve several health conditions, such as diabetes, Alzheimer's, Parkinson's, epilepsy, and even cancer.

A comparison of several scientific trials shows that low-carb diets outperform calorie-restricted diets in terms of long-term weight loss and lasting health effects. Restricting carbohydrates is a very effective way of controlling appetite, which explains why so many people successfully lose weight on a low-carb diet. Again, the key factor is insulin.

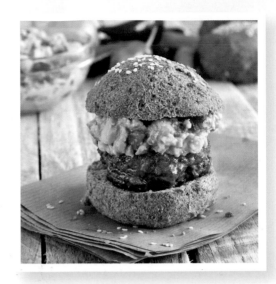

It's released when you eat carbs, and it affects your appetite: eating fewer carbs means you'll experience fewer cravings.

DO WE REALLY NEED CARBS?

A common misconception is that our bodies—especially our brains—need glucose. However, apart from some basic metabolic functions that need glucose exclusively, our bodies can use *either* glucose or ketones for energy: in fact, glucose is nowhere near as efficient as ketone bodies. Provided you eat enough protein, your body can produce glucose for its basic metabolic functions on demand via a process called *gluconeogenesis*, in which it transforms noncarbohydrate sources, such as amino acids (proteins) and fatty acids (fats), into glucose.

THE KETODIET APPROACH

The KetoDiet approach is simple: It's a low-carb diet with a focus on eating *real* food.

With the growing popularity of low-carb diets, the food industry introduced many new low-carb convenience foods. While such foods may indeed be low in carbs, they're often laden with unhealthy ingredients, such as artificial sweeteners, preservatives, and other additives. You won't find any of these things in my recipes—and you won't find grains, sugar, potatoes, legumes, or unhealthy oils in them, either. (But you will find dairy-free options in a number of my recipes.)

For the ketogenic diet to yield the best results, tracking your food intake is highly recommended, since it's very easy to go over your carb limit if you're new to this way of eating. My recipes contain detailed nutritional information so you can easily track your food intake, especially carbs. Ideally, you'll plan your daily meals in advance, and you'll be aware of all carbs you consume. Remember, it's not okay to have a piece of cake, a bag of chips, or a bowl of pasta—*especially* not at the beginning of the diet. Yes, it will be hard for the first couple of weeks, but the results will be more than rewarding!

THE BASIC PRINCIPLES

As you learn more about keto-friendly foods and get used to ketogenic/low-carb living, it'll be easier for you to understand what and how much you should be eating. Here's a crash course in what your daily macronutrient—carbs, protein, and fat—should look like.

Carbohydrates (5% to 10% of Your Daily Energy Requirements)

Each person's carb tolerance is different. Your challenge is to find your "ideal" carb intake. As you begin your KetoDiet, start with a low level of net carbs to ensure you quickly enter ketosis—the state in which your body produces ketone bodies. A good goal would be about 20 grams of net carbs per day. You can purchase a blood ketone meter (or urine ketone strips, which are less accurate) that will allow you to measure your ketones after about two or three days of sticking to your new low-carb lifestyle. Start adding net carbs (about 5 grams each week) until you detect a very low level of ketones or none at all. This is usually the quickest, most reliable way to discover your net carbs limit. You can find blood ketone meters and urine ketone strips via online retailers, such as Amazon.

Total Carbs or Net Carbs?

To follow a low-carb, ketogenic diet, you can limit either your total carb intake or your net carb intake. Net carbs are total carbs without fiber.

Most people who follow a ketogenic diet stay below 20 to 30 grams of net carbs or 50 grams of total carbs, as recommended by physicians Jeff Volek and Stephen Phinney, authors of *The Art and Science of Low Carbohydrate Living*. It's up to you which path you choose.

And, although some people fear that fiber raises blood sugar, recent studies show that fiber may actually reduce it.

Keto-Flu and the Importance of Electrolytes

No matter how old you are, your body is probably used to sugar and glucose at this point in your life. Excluding it from your diet may lead to headaches, weakness, or fatigue during the first few days of your new ketogenic lifestyle. These symptoms—sometimes referred to as "keto flu"—should dissipate after a few days or weeks. Increasing your intake of electrolytes (sodium, magnesium, and potassium) can minimize these negative side effects. Try my homemade Bone Broth (page 30) and eat foods high in electrolytes, such as avocados, nuts, fatty fish, dark leafy greens, spinach, and mushrooms.

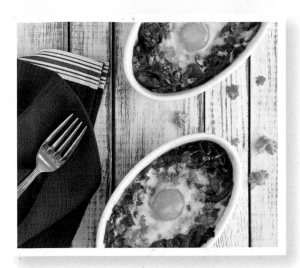

Make sure you eat at least the minimum amount of protein to prevent loss of muscle tissue during the diet. In general, the more active you are, the closer you should be eating to your upper limit.

Protein (15% to 30% of Your Daily Energy Requirements)

The amount of dietary protein you need can be determined by your body weight and activity level. People who are physically active have higher protein requirements than those with sedentary lifestyles. A more accurate estimate, especially for people with high body fat, can be reached by calculating protein intake from lean mass, which is calculated as total body weight minus body fat.

Eating enough protein is important for preserving and building muscle mass, but eating excessive amounts of protein is likely to put you out of ketosis because your body will convert excessive protein into glycogen.

How Many Grams of Protein per Day?

If your weight is in pounds, multiply it by 0.6 to get the minimum amount of protein in grams you should eat each day. For the maximum, multiply your body weight by 1 (i.e., the same numeral as that of your weight). If your weight is in kilograms, simply multiply it by 1.3 and 2.2 to get the same range. Although this rule applies to the majority of people, protein requirements for athletes are higher.

Fat (60% to 75% of Your Daily Energy Requirements)

Your daily fat intake should make up your remaining energy needs; it acts as "filler" for your energy requirements. Ideal fat intake varies for each individual and depends on your personal goal. In general, you won't need to precisely count fat intake or calories on a ketogenic diet, as you'll be unlikely to overeat: eating foods naturally low in carbs, moderate in protein, and high in fat will keep you satiated for longer. Studies have shown that protein and fats are the most satiating nutrients, while carbohydrates are the least satiating. Fat provides a steady supply of energy with no insulin spikes. That's why you won't experience any cravings or energy and mood swings as you would on a calorie-restricted, low-fat diet.

HEALTHY OILS AND FATS

Since you'll be increasing your fat intake, it's critical to understand which fats are beneficial and which may damage your health. Not all fats are created equal: simply put, the type and quality of fats matter. Follow these rules when you're choosing oils and fats:

- Use oils and fats high in saturated fats for all cooking (pure pastured lard, ghee, butter, grass-fed beef tallow, coconut oil, cacao butter, and red palm oil). Use extra virgin coconut oil, which is high in medium-chain triglycerides (MCTs) or try pure MCT oil for extra-effective fat-burning.

- Use oils and fats high in monounsaturated fats for light cooking and in salads (extra virgin olive oil, avocado oil, and macadamia nut oil).

- Use oils and fats high in polyunsaturated fats only in salads and for other cold uses. Oils high in polyunsaturated fats are nut and seed oils, like walnut, almond, hazelnut, flaxseed, or pumpkin seed oil. Increase your intake of omega-3 fatty acids, especially from animal sources, and avoid using too many oils high in omega-6 fatty acids (sesame oil, almond oil, etc.).

- Never use unhealthy fats like margarine, sunflower, rapeseed/canola, safflower, soy, cottonseeds, or grapeseed. All these are either processed, genetically-modified oils, or have a very unhealthy omega-6 to omega-3 ratio.

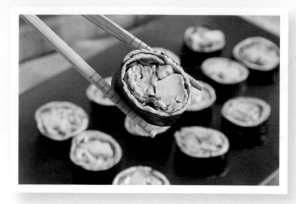

Do Calories Count?

Well, yes. It's a common misconception that you can eat an unlimited amount of calories and still lose weight. In fact, you can put on weight even on a low-carb diet. Although this doesn't happen often, understanding a few basic principles will help you avoid common mistakes.

Low-carb ketogenic diets are naturally satiating and act as appetite suppressants. This is why you'll eat less and won't need to count calories. However, if your weight is stalling for more than two to three weeks, you may need to consider keeping an eye on your energy intake.

That said, hitting a weight-loss plateau may be caused by a number of reasons. You don't necessarily have to be eating too much: in fact, you may discover that you haven't been eating enough. Avoiding sweeteners and abstaining from snacking between meals may also help you break through a plateau. And, in my experience, losing body fat becomes more difficult as you get closer to your target weight.

THE KETODIET A NUTSHELL

Here's a handy reference to use as you begin your new KetoDiet lifestyle:

- Stick with the keto ratio: 60% to 75% of calories from fat, 15% to 30% calories from protein, and 5% to 10% calories from net carbs.

- Get your daily net carbs (total carbs without fiber) down to less than 50 grams, preferably to 20 to 30 grams.

- Keep your protein intake moderate (0.6 to 1 g per pound, or 1.3 to 2.2 g per kilogram of lean body mass).

- Eat more healthy fats (saturated, omega 3s, and monounsaturated).

- Eat when you're hungry, even if it's only a meal a day. You don't have to limit quantities of food deliberately, but you should stop eating when you feel full.

- Don't count calories. Your diet will be naturally satiating.

- Drink more water.

- Beware of hidden carbs and unhealthy ingredients. Always read the labels.

- Avoid eating anything labeled "low-fat" or "fat-free." Focus on eating real food, like meat, eggs, nonstarchy vegetables, and whole dairy.

- Don't trust products labeled "low-carb." Instead, focus on foods that are naturally low in carbs.

- Up your electrolytes (sodium, magnesium, and potassium). Include avocados, nuts, and leafy greens in your diet. Take supplements if needed.

- Be prepared: plan your diet in advance to avoid "accidents." Keep motivated and focus on your targets!

THE KETODIET FOOD LIST

Use the following information as your guidelines for healthy eating on the KetoDiet.

Eat Freely

Grass-Fed and Wild Animal Sources

- grass-fed meat (beef, lamb, goat, and venison): Avoid sausages and meat covered in breadcrumbs, hot dogs, and meat that comes with sugary or starchy sauces.

- wild-caught fish and seafood

- pastured pork and poultry

- pastured eggs

- gelatin

- ghee and butter

- offal, grass-fed (liver, heart, kidneys, and other organ meats)

Healthy Fats

- saturated (pure pastured lard, grass-fed beef tallow, chicken fat, duck fat, goose fat, clarified butter/ghee, butter, and coconut oil)

- monounsaturated (avocado, macadamia, and olive oil)

- polyunsaturated omega 3s, especially from animal sources (fatty fish and seafood)

Nonstarchy Vegetables

- leafy greens (Swiss chard, bok choy, spinach, lettuce, chard, chives, endive, radicchio, etc.)

- some cruciferous vegetables (kale, kohlrabi, and radishes)

- celery stalks, asparagus, cucumber, summer squash, zucchini, spaghetti squash, and bamboo shoots

Fruits, Nuts, and Seeds

- avocado

- coconut

- macadamia nuts

Beverages and Condiments

- water, coffee (black or with cream or coconut milk), tea (black or herbal)
- pork rinds (cracklings) for "breading"
- mayonnaise, mustard, pesto, bone broth, pickles, and fermented foods (kimchi, kombucha, and sauerkraut)—best when they're homemade with no additives
- all spices and herbs, and lemon or lime juice and zest
- whey protein (beware of additives, artificial sweeteners, hormones, and soy lecithin), egg white protein, and gelatin (grass-fed, hormone-free)

Eat Occasionally

Vegetables, Mushrooms, and Fruits

- some cruciferous vegetables (white and green cabbage, red cabbage, cauliflower, broccoli, brussels sprouts, fennel, turnips, and rutabaga)
- nightshades (eggplant, tomatoes, and peppers)
- some root vegetables (parsley root), spring onion, leek, onion, garlic, mushrooms, and winter squash (pumpkin)
- sea vegetables (nori and kombu), okra, bean sprouts, sugar snap peas, wax beans, globe or French artichokes, and water chestnuts
- berries (blackberries, blueberries, strawberries, raspberries, cranberries, mulberries, etc.), rhubarb, and olives

Grain-Fed Animal Sources and Dairy

- beef, poultry, eggs, and ghee
- dairy products (plain full-fat yogurt, cottage cheese, cream, sour cream, and cheese): Avoid products labeled "low-fat," as most are packed with sugar and starch and have little satiating effect.
- bacon: Beware of preservatives and added starches.

Nuts and Seeds

- pecans, almonds, walnuts, hazelnuts, pine nuts, flaxseed, pumpkin seeds, sesame seeds, sunflower seeds, and hemp seeds
- brazil nuts (avoid overeating, due to their high selenium levels)

Fermented Soy Products

- non-GMO, fermented soy products only (natto, tempeh, soy sauce, or paleo-friendly coconut aminos)
- edamame (green soy beans) and black soybeans—unprocessed

Condiments

- healthy "zero-carb" sweeteners (stevia, Swerve, erythritol, etc.)
- thickeners: arrowroot powder, xanthan gum (technically, xanthan gum isn't paleo-friendly, but some people following the paleo diet use it since most recipes only call for a very small amount)
- sugar-free tomato products (puree, pasta sauce, and ketchup)
- cacao and carob powder, extra dark chocolate (more than 70% cocoa: 90% is better), and cacao powder
- Beware of "sugar-free" chewing gums and mints which contain carbs.

Some Vegetables, Fruits, Nuts, and Seeds with Average Carbohydrates

- root vegetables (celery root, carrot, beetroot, parsnip, and sweet potato)
- apricot, watermelon, cantaloupe/galia/honeydew melons, dragon fruit (pitaya), peach, nectarine, apple, grapefruit, kiwifruit, kiwi berries, orange, plums, cherries, pears, and figs (fresh)
- dried fruit (dates, berries, raisins, figs, etc.)—only in very small quantities (if any)
- pistachio and cashew nuts and chestnuts

Alcohol
- dry red wine, dry white wine, and spirits (unsweetened): avoid for weight loss and use only during weight maintenance

Avoid Completely
Food Rich in Carbohydrates, Factory-Farmed Meat, and Processed Foods
- all grains, even whole meal (wheat, rye, oats, corn, barley, millet, bulgur, sorghum, rice, amaranth, buckwheat, and sprouted grains), quinoa, and potatoes: This includes all products made from grains (pasta, bread, pizza, cookies, crackers, etc.).
- sugar and sweets (table sugar, high-fructose corn syrup, agave syrup, ice creams, cakes, sweet puddings, and sugary soft-drinks)
- factory-farmed pork and fish, which are high in inflammatory omega-6 fatty acids: farmed fish may contain polychlorinated biphenyls (PCBs)
- fish that are high in mercury (swordfish, king mackerel, shark, etc.)
- processed foods containing carrageenan (e.g., almond milk products), MSG (e.g., some whey protein products), sulphites (e.g., dried fruits, gelatin), or PCBs (e.g., in some farmed fish): They don't always appear on the label!
- artificial sweeteners (Splenda, Equal, sweeteners containing aspartame, acesulfame, sucralose, saccharin, etc.)
- refined fats/oils (e.g., sunflower, safflower, cottonseed, canola, soybean, grapeseed, and corn oil) and trans fats such as margarine
- "low-fat," "low-carb," and "zero-carb" products (Atkins products, diet soda and drinks, chewing gums, and mints may be high in carbs or contain artificial additives, gluten, etc.)

- milk (only small amounts of raw, full-fat milk is allowed. Milk is not recommended for several reasons. Of all dairy products, milk is most difficult to digest, as it lacks the "good" bacteria—eliminated through pasteurization—and may even contain hormones, and it is quite high in carbs [4 to 5 grams of carbs per 100 ml]. For coffee and tea, replace milk with cream in reasonable amounts. You may have a small amount of raw milk, but be aware of the extra carbs.)
- alcoholic and sweet drinks (beer, sweet wine, cocktails, etc.), apart from small amounts of spirits and dry wine
- tropical fruit (pineapple, mango, banana, papaya, etc.) and some high-carb fruit (tangerine, grapes, etc.). Avoid fruit juices (yes, even 100% fresh juices!); smoothies are better, since they have fiber, but they too should be limited. This also includes dried fruit (dates, raisins, etc.) if eaten in large quantities.
- Soy products, apart from a few non-GMO fermented products that are known for their health benefits
- Wheat gluten, which may be used in some low-carb foods
- Products containing BPA: Beware of BPA-lined cans. If possible, use naturally BPA-free packaging, like glass jars, or make your own ingredients, such as ghee, ketchup, coconut milk, or mayonnaise. BPA has been linked to many negative health effects, such as impaired thyroid function and cancer.

Suitable Low-Carb Sweeteners

Figuring out which sweeteners are appropriate for a ketogenic or other low-carb diet can be confusing. First of all, avoiding sugar completely is critical for succeeding at the ketogenic lifestyle. Second, not all sweeteners are suitable for a low-carb diet, and not all low-carb sweeteners are healthy.

So what about "healthy" sweeteners? Raw honey, blackstrap molasses, date syrup, rice malt syrup, maple syrup, or coconut palm sugar are often recommended on a paleo diet. However, if your aim is to lose weight, you should avoid them. Sugar is sugar. No matter how healthy the sweetener is, it will always impair your weight loss and can potentially kick you out of ketosis. Here's a list of the best keto-friendly sweeteners:

Stevia

Stevia is one of the best low-carb sweeteners, and it's my personal favorite. The extract is made from the herb stevia, and it has no calories and no effect on blood sugar. I use stevia drops for the recipes in this book, but you can use powdered stevia instead. The sweetness of products containing stevia varies, so you'll have to adjust them to your palate: keep in mind that stevia drops are about 200 to 300 times sweeter than sugar. And remember that too much stevia will make the final result bitter, so combine stevia with erythritol or Swerve to avoid any unpleasant aftertaste. (As always, make sure you avoid sweeteners with added sugar, dextrose, and maltodextrin, which will spike your blood sugar levels.)

Erythritol and Swerve

Erythritol is naturally found in fruits, vegetables, and fermented foods. It is a sugar alcohol that does not affect blood glucose and has very few calories. Erythritol is commonly used in low-carb cooking, and it's one of my favorites: I often combine it with liquid stevia. Some of the recipes in this book ask you to powder erythritol before mixing with other ingredients: that's because erythritol remains grainy unless it's heated. Swerve is an erythritol-based sweetener that is great for low-carb baking.

Monk Fruit Powder

This sweetener is also known as lo han or luo han. It's as sweet as stevia, but without the bitter aftertaste of most stevia products. Sweeteners containing monk fruit extract may contain other ingredients: keep that in mind and avoid any sweeteners with added sugar, artificial sweeteners, dextrose, or maltodextrin.

Xylitol

Xylitol is a sugar alcohol that naturally occurs in the fibers of certain fruits and vegetables. It's a sugar substitute that tastes like sugar but has fewer calories. Xylitol has a glycemic index of 13 and has 3 calories per gram. It does not affect blood sugar significantly if consumed in moderation. However, Xylitol may cause digestive issues in some people, especially if you eat more than 50 grams.

Inulin-Based Sweeteners

Chicory root inulin (chicory root fiber) is probably the most popular inulin-based sweetener. Inulin has been shown to have health-promoting prebiotic effects. Some of the inulin-type prebiotics are called fructooligosaccharides (FOS), which are a type of carbohydrate that our bodies cannot fully digest. Consumption of FOS does not increase blood sugar.

Yacon Syrup

Yacon syrup has a slightly caramel taste and is similar to blackstrap molasses and coconut palm sugar. It consists of 50% FOS and a fiber called inulin that doesn't increase blood sugar. However, because it does have a small effect on blood sugar, you should use it very sparingly.

Sweeteners to Avoid

Avoid all sweeteners containing carbs, such as table sugar, high-fructose corn syrup, and agave syrup. Agave syrup may be sold as a "health" food, but the truth is, it's loaded with unhealthy fructose. Artificial sweeteners like aspartame, saccharin, sucralose, or acesulfame K may seem like an ideal option while following a healthy low-carb diet, but you should avoid them: Not only do they cause sugar cravings, but regular consumption of them is also linked to several negative health effects such as bloating, migraines, and weight gain. Some are even linked to certain types of cancer.

Cooking Ketogenic

When you're sourcing ingredients, try to get them in their most natural forms: that is, organically grown and free from unnecessary additives. Buy organic eggs; organic unwaxed lemons; pastured beef and butter; outdoor-reared pork; wild-caught fish; and extra virgin coconut oil.

Remember:

- All the recipes in this book are well-suited to the ketogenic, paleo, and primal diets. Additionally, several recipes include dairy-free options.

- Nutrition values for each recipe are per serving unless stated otherwise. The nutrition data are derived from the USDA National Nutrient Database (http://ndb.nal.usda.gov).

- Nutrition facts are calculated from edible parts. For example, if one avocado is listed as 200 g/7.1 oz, this value represents its edible parts (seeds and peel removed) unless otherwise specified.

- Optional ingredients and suggestions are not included in the nutrition information.

AN IMPORTANT NOTE ABOUT MEASUREMENTS

If you are following a ketogenic diet for specific health reasons, you should be aware that accuracy is vital for this diet to work. When measuring ingredients, always weigh them using a kitchen scale. Using measures like cups or tablespoons can lead to inaccuracies that may impact the macronutrient composition of your meal. All it takes to shift your body out of ketosis is a few extra grams of carbohydrates. Furthermore, cups and tablespoons for dried products (psyllium, flax meal, etc.) may vary depending on the brand. Using a less-than-precise amount of an ingredient will affect the quality of a recipe—particularly for baked goods—and the final result will be less than desirable.

Chapter Two:

HOMEMADE BASICS

Starting a low-carb diet often means giving up your favorite comfort foods—especially baked or starchy items like tortillas and buns. That's why I decided to create healthy, low-carb alternatives to some of these popular foods. In this chapter, you'll learn how to make delicious, satisfying breads, buns, pancakes, and tortillas that can be enjoyed on their own, or combined with other sweet or savory ingredients to make a meal. Plus, you'll find out how to make homemade versions of common condiments—healthy versions of the "stealth" ingredients that can ruin a low-carb diet. Making your own mayonnaise, ketchup, or mustard will help you avoid the unhealthy sugar and additives that often turn up in popular products. (And they taste better than the store-bought, stuff, too!)

ULTIMATE KETO BREAD

My Ultimate Keto Bread is one of the best low-carb breads you'll ever try.
It's high in heart-healthy monounsaturated fats, and it's lovely
topped with grass-fed butter!

1 LOAF/12 SLICES	15 MINS	1 HOUR 15 MINS

INGREDIENTS

Dry Ingredients

5.3 ounces (150 g) macadamia nuts

¼ cup (30 g/1.1 oz) coconut flour

½ cup (50 g/1.8 oz) whey protein or pastured egg white protein powder, unflavored

⅔ cup (80 g/2.8 oz) psyllium husk powder

1 teaspoon baking soda

2 teaspoons cream of tartar

1 teaspoon salt

Wet Ingredients

4 large pastured eggs, whole

2 large pastured egg whites

1 cup (240 ml/8 fl oz) water, room temperature

NUTRITION FACTS PER SERVING

Total carbs: 8.2 g

Fiber: 6.3 g

Net carbs: 1.9 g

Protein: 7.6 g

Fat: 11.5 g

Energy: 143 kcal

Macronutrient ratio: Calories from carbs (6%), protein (21%), fat (73%)

Preheat the oven to 350°F (175°C, or gas mark 4). Line a large loaf pan (about 7 × 4½ inches/18 × 12 cm) with parchment paper or use a silicone loaf pan. Grind the macadamia nuts using an electric or manual nut grinder. (If you don't have macadamia nuts, use an equal amount of almond flour and add an extra ¼ cup [60 ml/2 fl oz] of water to the wet ingredients.)

Mix all the dry ingredients apart from the cream of tartar in a medium bowl. (Do not use whole psyllium husks; if you can't find psyllium husk powder, process the husks in a blender or coffee grinder until finely ground.)

Crack the eggs and place the egg whites and egg yolks into separate bowls. Mix the egg yolks with the water until well combined. Beat all six egg whites until they create soft (not too firm) peaks. Add the cream of tartar throughout the whisking process.

Add the dry ingredients to the egg yolk mixture. Add the whisked egg whites and mix well: you don't need to be too gentle, but try not to deflate them completely. Whisked egg whites incorporate better than whole whites.

Transfer the dough into the parchment paper-lined loaf pan. Place in the oven and bake for about 60 minutes. To test for doneness, insert a long wooden skewer into the bread. If there are no crumbs on it and it comes out clean, the bread is done. If you're using a regular loaf pan with parchment paper, remove the loaf from the pan by pulling on the parchment paper: this will help prevent excess moisture from accumulating on the outside of the loaf. Let cool before slicing. Store covered with a kitchen towel for up to 3 days or freeze in an airtight container for longer.

FLUFFY GRAIN-FREE SUNFLOWER BREAD

Wonderfully fluffy and light, this Sunflower Bread is great with nut butter, cream cheese, butter, or my Spiced Berry Jam (page 40).

1 LOAF/12 SLICES	15 MINS	1 HOUR 15 MINS

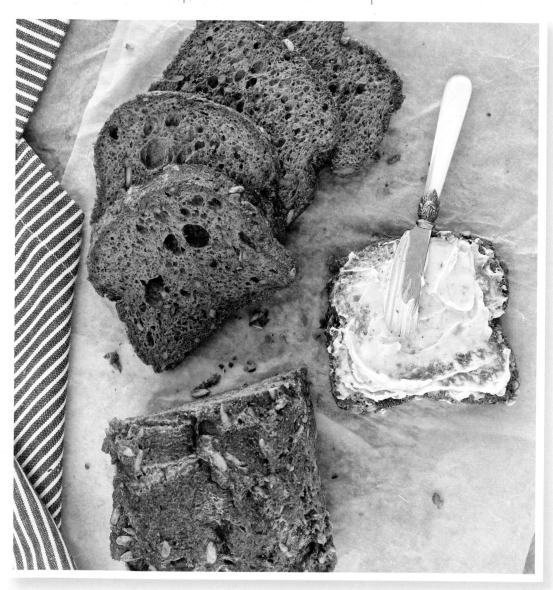

INGREDIENTS

Wet Ingredients

4 large pastured eggs, whole

2 large pastured egg whites

2 tablespoons (30 ml/1 fl oz) toasted sesame oil

2 tablespoons (30 g/1.1 oz) ghee or butter

½ cup (120 ml/4 fl oz) water, at room temperature

DRY INGREDIENTS

¼ cup (40 g/1.4 oz) flax meal

⅔ cup (80 g/2.8 oz) psyllium husk powder

1 teaspoon baking soda

1 tablespoon (7 g/0.2 oz) caraway seeds

1 teaspoon salt

2 teaspoons cream of tartar

½ cup (70 g/2.5 oz) sunflower seeds

NUTRITION FACTS PER SLICE

Total carbs: 8 g

Fiber: 6.4 g

Net carbs: 1.6 g

Protein: 4.8 g

Fat: 10.7 g

Energy: 124 kcal

Macronutrient ratio: Calories from carbs (5%), protein (16%), fat (79%)

Preheat the oven to 350°F (175°C, or gas mark 4). Line a large loaf pan (about 7 × 4.5 inch/18 × 12 cm) with parchment paper or use a silicone loaf pan. Working with the wet ingredients first, separate the egg yolks from the egg whites. Set the egg whites aside in a bowl.

Mix the egg yolks with the toasted sesame oil and melted ghee or butter. Pour the water into the egg yolk mixture and combine well.

In a separate bowl, mix the flax meal, psyllium husk powder, baking soda, caraway seeds, and salt. (Do not use whole psyllium husks; if you can't find psyllium husk powder, process the husks in a blender or coffee grinder until finely ground.)

Beat the egg whites until they create soft peaks. Add the cream of tartar while beating; this helps the egg whites stay fluffy.

Using an electric mixer, add the egg yolk mixture to the bowl with the dry ingredients and process well. Slowly add the whisked egg whites: you don't need to be too gentle, but try not to deflate them completely.

Fold the sunflower seeds into the batter. Fill the loaf pan with the batter and transfer to the oven. Bake for about 60 minutes. To test for doneness, insert a long wooden skewer into the bread. If there are no crumbs on it and it comes out clean, the bread is done.

If you're using a regular loaf pan with parchment paper, remove the loaf from the pan by pulling on the parchment paper: this will help prevent excess moisture from accumulating on the outside of the loaf. Let the loaf cool on a tray for at least 15 to 20 minutes. Store at room temperature covered with a kitchen towel for up to three days or place in a zip-top bag and freeze for longer.

TIPS

- Make sure you follow the recipe step by step. Even a small change can result in a lumpy texture or a batter that's too moist. If you don't add the water into the egg yolks and do so separately after you mix in the egg yolks, the texture will become lumpy and rubbery.

- If your bread turns out to be a vibrant green color, don't panic—it's perfectly safe. Sunflower seeds contain chlorogenic acid, an antioxidant that gives the seeds the ability to turn green when mixed with alkaline baking ingredients like baking soda.

LOW-CARB SOURDOUGH BREAD

It took me weeks of fine-tuning to come up with the perfect recipe for a low-carb sourdough bread, but all my hard work paid off! It's not as crispy as regular sourdough, but toasting it before serving makes it absolutely delicious.

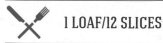 1 LOAF/12 SLICES | 15 MINS | 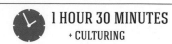 1 HOUR 30 MINUTES + CULTURING

INGREDIENTS

Culturing Ingredients

10.6 ounces (300 g) macadamia nuts

½ cup (120 ml/4 fl oz) water

As many probiotic capsules as you need to get 30 to 40 billion live probiotic cultures (about 16 capsules)

Dry Ingredients

⅔ cup (80 g/2.8 oz) psyllium husk powder

¾ cup (75 g/2.6 oz) almond flour

¼ cup (30g/1.1 oz) coconut flour

1 teaspoon baking soda

1 teaspoon salt

2 teaspoons cream of tartar

Wet Ingredients

5 large pastured eggs, whole

1 large pastured egg white

½ cup (120 ml/4 fl oz) water

Put the macadamias and water into a blender. Pulse until very smooth. The mixture should be quite thick; do not add more water. (If you don't have macadamia nuts, use the same amount of ground blanched almonds.)

Pour the blended nuts into a bowl. Open each probiotic capsule one by one and add the powder from each to the bowl. Mix until well combined. I like my bread sour, so I used 16 capsules with 2.5 billion live cultures in each. The more capsules you use, the more sour the dough will be.

Set a plate on top of the bowl and transfer to the oven. Turn the oven light on. This should be enough to slowly bring the temperature to 105 to 110°F (40 to 45°C)—the perfect conditions for culturing the macadamia nuts. Don't turn the oven on if you don't have to; just use the light. If the temperature is too high, it will kill the bacteria and it won't culture: if the temperature is too low, it will culture slowly or not at all. Alternatively, you can also use a food dehydrator or a yogurt maker.

After 12 to 24 hours (the longer you leave it, the more sour the dough will be), remove the dough from the oven. Preheat the oven to 350°F (175°C, or gas mark 4). Line a large loaf pan (about 7 × 4.5 inch/18 × 12 cm) with parchment paper or use a silicone loaf pan.

Combine the psyllium husk powder, almond flour, coconut flour, baking soda, and salt in a separate bowl and mix well.

Total carbs: 11.2 g

Fiber: 8.2 g

Net carbs: 3.1 g

Protein: 6.9 g

Fat: 24.6 g

Energy: 264 kcal

Macronutrient ratio: Calories from carbs (5%), protein (10%), fat (85%)

Separate all the egg yolks from the egg whites and place in two bowls. (You will need a total of 4 mixing bowls for this recipe: one for the egg yolks, one for egg whites, one for the dry mixture, and one for the macadamia nut mixture.) Set one egg yolk aside; you will brush the top of the bread with it. You'll have one egg yolk left over, which you can use in another recipe. Add the remaining water to the bowl with the 4 egg yolks and mix well.

Beat the egg whites until they create soft peaks, gradually adding the cream of tartar throughout the process. When done, set it aside. Pour the egg yolk mixture into the dry mixture and combine well (an electric blender is ideal).

Add the cultured macadamia nut dough and process well. Add the whisked egg whites and mix until well combined. You don't need to be too gentle but try not to deflate the whites completely; use a slow blending option.

Transfer the dough into the pan lined with parchment paper or use a silicone loaf pan. Brush the top of the dough with the reserved egg yolk. (If the egg yolk is too thick or dry, mix it with a teaspoon of water.) This egg wash will give your bread a crispy, golden finish. Bake for about 60 minutes.

When done, the top should be rounded and golden in color. (Note: If you use a pan that's too large, you may not get a rounded top.) Store at room temperature covered with a kitchen towel for up to three days or place in a zip-top bag and freeze for longer.

TIP

Make sure you follow this recipe step by step: even a small change can result in failure. Here's one of my most memorable failed experiments: When I cultured all the ingredients together (macadamia nuts, almond flour, coconut flour, and psyllium) instead of adding the dry ingredients just before baking, the bread looked unappetizing and had a jelly texture. (Yuck!) Also, be careful not to use extra water. If you do, the dough will be too moist and won't rise properly.

ESSENTIAL KETO CREPES

*They feel festive and fancy, but crepes are so quick and easy—
and they can be either savory or sweet, depending on your mood.
You can also use them in place of tortillas or wraps.*

 4 SERVINGS | **5 MINS** | **15 MINS**

INGREDIENTS

2 large eggs

6 large egg whites

2 tablespoons (24 g/0.8 oz) coconut flour

1 tablespoon (8 g/0.3 oz) psyllium husk powder or ground chia seeds

¼ cup plus 2 tablespoons (90 ml/3 fl oz) coconut milk, cream or almond milk

½ teaspoon gluten-free baking soda

1 teaspoon cream of tartar

2 tablespoons (30 g/1.1 oz) ghee or coconut oil

2 teaspoons garlic powder or onion powder

Salt to taste

NUTRITION FACTS PER SERVING

Total carbs: 5.5 g

Fiber: 2.6 g

Net carbs: 2.9 g

Protein: 10.2 g

Fat: 19.4 g

Energy: 239 kcal

Macronutrient ratio: Calories from carbs (5%), protein (18%), fat (77%)

Separate the egg whites from the egg yolks. You will only need 2 egg yolks and 8 egg whites, as the crepes hold better together when more egg whites are used. Reserve any remaining egg yolks for use in another recipe.

Place the whole eggs and egg whites, coconut flour, psyllium husk powder or chia seeds, coconut milk, baking soda, and cream of tartar in a bowl and mix well. (You can use heavy whipping cream or almond milk in place of the coconut milk, if you like: these have less carbs and fat.)

Add the garlic powder and whisk well. Alternatively, to make sweet crepes, use a few drops of stevia or 2 tablespoons (20 g) of erythritol in place of the garlic powder.

Let the batter sit for 5 to 10 minutes so the coconut flour and psyllium have time to soak up the moisture. Then whisk again. Add water if the mixture is too thick. (If you can't find psyllium husk powder, process the husks in a blender or coffee grinder until finely ground.)

Heat a nonstick pan evenly greased with ghee over a medium heat. Move the pan while pouring the batter in to ensure that the mixture covers the bottom of the pan in a thin layer. The batter should be runny so that you can spread it easily. If it's too thick, add a tablespoon (15 ml/0.5 fl oz) of water. Make the crepes one by one, greasing the pan in between with a small amount of oil to avoid sticking. Depending on the size of the crepes, you will get two large or four medium crepes per recipe. Use as wraps for meat and vegetables. Let cool and then store in an airtight container in the fridge for up to 5 days.

GRAIN-FREE TORTILLAS

Tortillas can easily be made crispy or soft, depending on cooking time. Wrap these beauties around some meat and vegetables and add dressing for a satisfying meal.

 10 SERVINGS | 20 MINS | 1 HOUR

INGREDIENTS

Dry Ingredients

1 cup (100 g/3.5 oz) almond flour

¾ cup (110 g/4 oz) flax meal

¼ cup (30 g/1.1 oz) coconut flour

2 tablespoons (8 g/0.3 oz) psyllium husks, whole

2 tablespoons (16 g/0.6 oz) chia seeds, ground

1 teaspoon garlic powder or onion powder

1 teaspoon salt

Wet Ingredients

1 cup (240 ml/8 fl oz) lukewarm water

2 tablespoons (30 g/1.1 oz) lard or ghee

NUTRITION FACTS PER SERVING

Total carbs: 7.4 g

Fiber: 5.7 g

Net carbs: 1.7 g

Protein: 5 g

Fat: 13.8 g

Energy: 165 kcal

Macronutrient ratio: Calories from carbs (5%), protein (13%), fat (82%)

Combine all the dry ingredients in a bowl and pour in one cup (240 ml/8 fl oz) of water. (If the dough is too dry to roll, add a few more tablespoons [45 to 60 ml/1.5 to 2 fl oz] of water. If you use too much, the dough will get too sticky and will become difficult to roll.) Mix well using your hands and shape into an oval. Let the dough rest in the fridge for up to an hour.

When ready, remove the dough from the fridge and cut it into six equal pieces. (You will use the excess dough after cutting the tortillas, in the next step, to make the remaining four tortillas.) Place a piece of the dough between two pieces of parchment paper and roll it out until very thin. Alternatively, use a silicone roller and a silicone mat.

Remove the top parchment paper and press a large 8-inch (20 cm) lid into the dough (or use a piece of parchment paper cut into a round shape: just trace around it with your knife) to cut out the tortilla.

Repeat for the remaining pieces of dough. Add the cut-off excess dough to the last piece and create the remaining 4 tortillas from it. If you have any dough left over, simply roll it out and cut it into tortilla-chip shapes.

Grease a large pan with the ghee or lard and cook one tortilla at a time for 2 to 3 minutes on each side over a medium heat until lightly browned. Don't overcook it: it'll become too crispy. Once cool, store the tortillas in an airtight container for up to a week and reheat them in a dry pan if needed.

(Note: Make sure you use whole psyllium husks in this recipe. Unlike other bread recipes in this book, this one doesn't use psyllium husk powder: whole husks make the tortillas more compact and flexible.)

ULTIMATE KETO BUNS

Are you missing "regular" bread? Never fear: these are the best low-carb buns you can imagine. They're nice and fluffy, and they taste just like the real thing!

 10 SERVINGS | 10 MINS | 1 HOUR

INGREDIENTS

Dry Ingredients

1½ cups (150 g/5.3 oz) almond flour

⅓ cup (40 g/2.8 oz) psyllium husk powder

½ cup (60 g/2.1 oz) coconut flour

½ cup (75 g/2.7 oz) flax meal

2 teaspoons garlic powder

2 teaspoons onion powder

1 teaspoon baking soda

2 teaspoons cream of tartar

1 teaspoon salt

5 tablespoons (40 g/1.4 oz) sesame seeds (or poppy, sunflower, or caraway seeds)

Wet Ingredients

6 large pastured egg whites

2 large pastured eggs

2 cups (470 ml/16 fl oz) boiling water

Preheat the oven to 350°F (175°C, or gas mark 4). Mix all the dry ingredients except the sesame seeds in a bowl. (Do not use whole psyllium husks; if you can't find psyllium husk powder, process the husks in a blender or coffee grinder until finely ground.)

Mix the eggs and egg whites in a separate bowl. Add the egg mixture to the dry ingredients and add the boiling water. Process well in a mixer until the dough is thick.

Using a spoon, form the dough into buns of equal sizes and place them on a nonstick baking sheet or a baking sheet lined with parchment paper (you could even use small tart trays). The buns will grow as they bake, so make sure to leave some space between each.

Top each of the buns with a sprinkling of sesame seeds and press the seeds into the dough so they won't fall out. Transfer the buns to the oven and bake for about 45 minutes.

Remove from the oven, let the tray cool, and then transfer the buns to a rack until they cool to room temperature. Store at room temperature if you plan to use the buns in the next couple of days or freeze for future use. Try them alongside your favorite salad, or use them as buns for my Ultimate GuacBurger (page 156). You can also shape them into bagels to make Healthy Salmon Bagels (page 83).

NUTRITION FACTS PER SLICE

Total carbs: 12.4 g

Fiber: 8.1 g

Net carbs: 4.2 g

Protein: 10.1 g

Fat: 15.2 g

Energy: 208 kcal

Macronutrient ratio: Calories from carbs (9%), protein (21%), fat (70%)

TIPS

· Psyllium absorbs lots of water. When you're baking with psyllium, remember to drink enough water throughout the day to prevent constipation!

· To speed things up, you can mix all the dry ingredients ahead of time and store them in a zip-top bag. Label the bag with the number of servings. When you're ready to bake, just add the wet ingredients.

· Make sure you weigh all the ingredients using scales. Even small differences can affect the final result of this recipe.

· If your buns appear to have large hollow bubbles inside them, it may be due to the psyllium. Again, make sure you use powder, not whole husks.

· If your buns don't rise properly, try the recipe again using only egg whites and omit the egg yolks altogether.

· If the final result is too moist, do not reduce the water used in this recipe—if you do, the psyllium will clump. Instead, dry the buns in the oven on low, up to 210°F (100°C), for 30 to 60 minutes. If necessary, cut them in half and place in a toaster.

· Don't let the batter sit for too long: put the buns in the oven as soon as you've formed them.

· Most of the above tips apply to any recipes using psyllium husk powder.

· Cream of tartar and baking soda act as leavening agents. This is how it works: To get 2 teaspoons of gluten-free baking powder, combine ½ teaspoon of baking soda with 1 teaspoon of cream of tartar.

MAYONNAISE

Mayonnaise is a fantastic keto-friendly condiment. To ensure best results, be sure to set any refrigerated ingredients out on your countertop to let them reach room temperature before you begin.

ABOUT 1 CUP (240 G)	15 MINS	15 MINS

INGREDIENTS

1 pastured egg yolk

1 teaspoon Dijon Mustard (page 31)

¾ cup (180 ml/6 fl oz) mild olive oil (or macadamia, avocado, or walnut oil)

1 tablespoon (15 ml/0.5 fl oz) lemon juice

1 tablespoon (15 ml/0.5 fl oz) apple cider vinegar

¼ teaspoon salt

Optional: 3 to 5 drops liquid stevia

1 teaspoon garlic powder or onion powder

NUTRITION FACTS PER SERVING

(1 tablespoon/15 g)
Total carbs: 0.1 g

Fiber: 0 g

Net carbs: 0.1 g

Protein: 0.2 g

Fat: 12.5 g

Energy: 111 kcal

Macronutrient ratio: Calories from carbs (0 %), protein (1 %), fat (99 %)

When all ingredients have reached room temperature, separate the egg white from the egg yolk. (Reserve the egg white for another recipe.) Place the yolk and Dijon mustard into a bowl. Blend until well combined.

Using a food processor or hand whisk to mix as you go, start to drizzle in the oil very slowly.

Keep drizzling in the oil until the mixture starts to look more like the consistency of mayonnaise. Steadily pour the oil in until all of it is incorporated. Keep mixing until the mayo reaches the desired thickness. If it doesn't seem thick enough, add a bit more oil.

Add the lemon juice and vinegar—which will turn the color a light yellow—then season with salt. If it is too tart, add a few drops of liquid stevia and mix well. If you think the consistency is too thick, add a few drops of water. To boost the flavor, add a teaspoon of garlic or onion powder and mix until well combined.

Transfer the mayonnaise to a glass container and seal well. You can store it in the fridge for up to a week. If you want the mayonnaise to last several months, add a tablespoon or two (15 to 30 g/0.5 to 1 oz) of whey.

TIP

When using raw eggs: Due to the slight risk of *Salmonella* and other foodborne illnesses, you should use only fresh, clean, properly-refrigerated grade A or AA eggs with intact shells. Avoid contact between the yolks or whites and the shell. Prevent any risks by using eggs with pasteurized shells.

KETCHUP

Store-bought products often contain added sugar and preservatives.
But that doesn't mean you have to do away with your favorite condiments.
You'll be surprised at how easy it is to make ketchup at home!

ABOUT 1 CUP (240 G)	5 MINS	15 MINS

INGREDIENTS

1 small (60 g/2.1 oz) white onion, peeled and cut into small pieces

2 cloves garlic, peeled and chopped

1 cup (240 g/8.5 oz) tomato puree, unsweetened

¼ cup (60 ml/2 fl oz) apple cider vinegar

⅛ teaspoon allspice

⅛ teaspoon ground cloves

3 to 6 drops liquid stevia

2 tablespoons (20 g/0.7 oz) erythritol or Swerve

1 teaspoon salt

Freshly ground black pepper to taste

¼ cup (60 ml/2 fl oz) water

NUTRITION FACTS PER SERVING

(1 tablespoon/15 g)

Total carbs: 1 g

Fiber: 0.2 g

Net carbs: 0.8 g

Protein: 0.2 g

Fat: 0 g

Energy: 4.8 kcal

Macronutrient ratio: Calories from carbs (77%), protein (7%), fat (6%)

Combine all the ingredients in a small saucepan and simmer, covered, over low heat for 5 to 10 minutes. Add a splash of water if the mixture seems too thick. When done, transfer the mixture to a blender and pulse until smooth. Pour the ketchup into a glass jar and store in the fridge for up to a month.

TIP

Homemade ketchup is a key ingredient in many other sauces, dressings, and dips, like my Spicy Chocolate BBQ Sauce (page 34)!

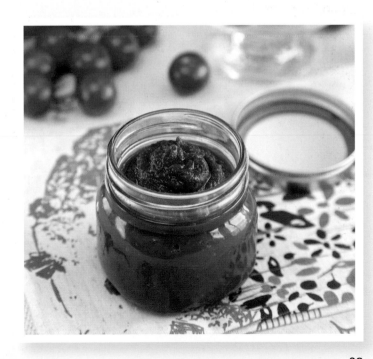

BONE BROTH

Drinking bone broth is one of the best ways to replenish electrolytes (sodium, magnesium, and potassium) and to eliminate the symptoms of keto-flu.

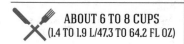

ABOUT 6 TO 8 CUPS (1.4 TO 1.9 L/47.3 TO 64.2 FL OZ)	10 MINS	🕐 2 HOURS OR MORE

INGREDIENTS

2 medium (120 g/4.2 oz) carrots

1 medium (90 g/3.2 oz) parsnip

1 medium (100 g/3.5 oz) white onion, peeled and halved

5 cloves garlic

2 (80 g/2.8 oz) celery stalks

3.3 pounds (1.5 kg) oxtail or assorted bones (chicken feet, marrowbones, etc.)

2 tablespoons (30 ml/1 fl oz) apple cider vinegar or lemon juice

2 to 3 bay leaves

1 tablespoon (18 g/0.6 oz) pink Himalayan or sea salt

8 to 10 cups (1.9 to 2.4 L/64 to 81 fl oz) water (enough to cover the bones, no more than ⅔ the capacity of the pressure cooker, ¾ the capacity of your Dutch oven, or ¾ the capacity of your slow cooker)

NUTRITION FACTS PER SERVING

(1 cup/235 ml/8 fl oz)

Total carbs: 0.9 g

Fiber: 0.2 g

Net carbs: 0.8 g

Protein: 3.6 g

Fat: 6 g

Energy: 72 kcal

Macronutrient ratio: Calories from carbs (4%), protein (20%), fat (76%)

Peel the carrots and parsnips and cut them into thirds. Halve the onion and peel and halve the garlic cloves. Keep the onion skin on to help the broth get a nice golden color. Wash and cut the celery into thirds. Place all of the ingredients into the pressure cooker or slow cooker.

In the pressure cooker: Lock the lid of your pressure cooker and turn it to high pressure/high heat. Once it reaches high pressure, turn it to the lowest heat and set the timer on the pressure cooker for 90 minutes. When done, take the pot off the heat and let the pressure release naturally for about 10 to 15 minutes before opening the lid. Pour the broth through a strainer into a large dish. Discard the vegetables and set the meaty bones aside to cool down. When the bones are chilled, shred the meat off with a fork. If there is any gelatin left on the bones, you can reuse them for another batch of Bone Broth: just store them in the freezer.

In the Dutch oven or slow cooker: Cover with a lid and cook for at least 6 hours on high or up to 48 hours on low. If you opt for longer cooking time, you'll have to remove the oxtail using tongs, shred the meat off using a fork, and then place the bones back into the pot.

Use the broth immediately or put it in the fridge overnight, where it will become partially jellied. Oxtail is high in fat, and the greasy layer on top—the tallow—will solidify. Simply scrape most of the tallow off and discard or reuse it for cooking. Keep the broth in the fridge if you're planning to use it over the next five days. For future uses, store it in small containers and freeze.

DIJON MUSTARD

Making mustard at home is so simple—and so rewarding.
It takes just a few minutes to prepare, and it tastes
amazing after a few weeks of aging in the fridge.

ABOUT 2 CUPS (480 G/16.9 OZ)	10 MINS	15 TO 20 MINS

INGREDIENTS

1 medium (110 g/3.9 oz) onion

2 cloves garlic

1 cup (240 ml/8 fl oz) dry white wine

¼ cup (60 ml/2 fl oz) white wine vinegar; or substitute with ¼ cup (60 ml/2 fl oz) vinegar and ¾ cup (180 ml/6 fl oz) of water

½ cup (120 ml/4 fl oz) water

1 cup (120 g/4.2 oz) mustard powder/ground mustard seeds

1 teaspoon ground turmeric

3 to 5 dashes Tabasco or other sugar-free hot sauce

5 to 10 drops liquid stevia

2 tablespoons (30 ml/1 fl oz) extra virgin olive oil (or macadamia, or avocado oil)

1 teaspoon salt

NUTRITION FACTS
PER SERVING

(1 tablespoon/15 g/0.5 oz)

Total carbs: 1.1 g

Fiber: 0.4 g

Net carbs: 0.7 g

Protein: 0.8 g

Fat: 1.7 g

Energy: 27 kcal

Macronutrient ratio: Calories from carbs (13%), protein (15%), fat (72%)

Peel and roughly chop the onion and garlic and place them in a nonreactive saucepan (see below). Pour in the wine, vinegar, and water and bring to a boil over medium heat. Simmer for about 5 minutes.

Cool and strain the mixture, discarding the solids. Place the mustard powder into a saucepan and add the strained liquid. Mix until well combined. Cook over low-medium heat until it thickens, about 2 to 5 minutes. Add the turmeric, Tabasco, stevia, oil, and salt.

Mix until well combined. Store in a jar in the refrigerator for up to 6 months. The mustard will taste best after a few weeks of aging.

TIP

You can make different types of mustard by adding a variety of optional ingredients. Try horseradish, fresh herbs, or whole grain mustard seeds.

WHAT IS A NONREACTIVE SAUCEPAN?

It's a saucepan made of a material that will not react with acidic ingredients. For example, stainless steel is nonreactive, while copper is a reactive material that will easily wear off if used with acidic ingredients like lemon juice or vinegar.

HOLLANDAISE SAUCE

Hollandaise sauce is easy. It's also the best way to add healthy fats to your diet and use up leftover egg yolks.

1 SERVING	10 MINS	10 MINS

INGREDIENTS

2 tablespoons (30 g/1.1 oz) butter

1 large pastured egg yolk

½ to 1 tablespoon (7.5 to 15 ml/0.25 to 0.5 fl oz) water, plus 1 cup (235 ml/8 fl oz) for steaming

1 tablespoon (15 ml/0.5 fl oz) lemon juice

¼ teaspoon Dijon mustard

Pinch of salt

NUTRITION FACTS PER SERVING

Total carbs: 1.5 g

Fiber: 0 g

Net carbs: 1.5 g

Protein: 3.1 g

Fat: 29 g

Energy: 274 kcal

Macronutrient ratio: Calories from carbs (2%), protein (4%), fat (94%)

Gently melt the butter and set aside; it should be warm, but not too hot. Mix the egg yolk with ½ to 1 tablespoon (7.5 to 15 ml/0.25 to 0.5 fl oz) of water, plus the lemon juice, Dijon mustard, and salt. Add the remaining water to a medium saucepan and bring to a boil. Keep it on medium heat. Place the bowl with the egg yolk mixture on top of the saucepan and stir continually. (For this to work, the bowl must be bigger than the saucepan, and the boiling water shouldn't reach the bottom of the bowl; only the steam heats the bowl.) Keep mixing until the mixture starts to thicken: then, very slowly, pour in the melted butter until it becomes thick and creamy. Stir constantly to avoid clumping. If the Hollandaise is too thick, add a splash of water. Serve immediately over poached eggs or baked salmon. Do not reheat the Hollandaise: it will clump. If you're making it only for yourself, prepare a single serving at a time.

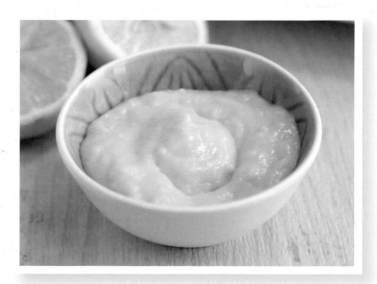

MARINARA SAUCE

This easy sauce can be used for pizza topping, with zucchini noodles, as a dip with fresh vegetables, or on low-carb bread.

	2 CUPS (490 G/17.3 OZ)		5 MINS		5 MINS

Wash and drain the tomatoes and basil. Peel the garlic and shallot. Add all the ingredients to a food processor and process until smooth. If you prefer a chunky texture, leave some tomatoes and basil aside to dice and add to the smooth sauce after it's blended. When done, store in an airtight container in the fridge for up to a week.

INGREDIENTS

1 cup (150 g/5.3 oz) cherry tomatoes

½ cup (20 g/0.7 oz) fresh basil

2 cloves garlic

1 small (30 g/1.1 oz) shallot

4 tablespoons (60 g/2.2 oz) tomato puree

¼ cup (60 ml/2 fl oz) extra virgin olive oil

¼ teaspoon salt

Freshly ground pepper

NUTRITION FACTS PER SERVING
(¼ cup/60 g/2.1 oz)

Total carbs: 3.5 g

Fiber: 0.8 g

Net carbs: 2.6 g

Protein: 0.7 g

Fat: 9.8 g

Energy: 101 kcal

Macronutrient ratio: Calories from carbs (10%), protein (3%), fat (87%)

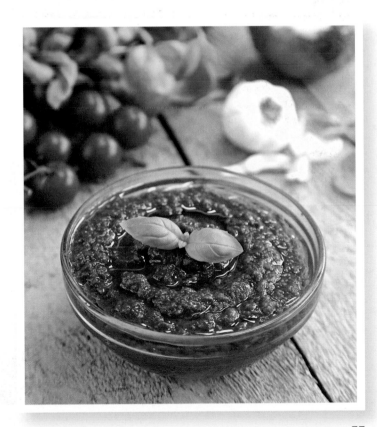

SPICY CHOCOLATE BBQ SAUCE

Are you bored with regular BBQ sauce? Try this sweet-and-spicy version, which can be used as a meat marinade or as a dip to accompany Zucchini Fries (see Sides).

1½ CUPS (375 G/13.2 OZ)	10 MINS	10 MINS

INGREDIENTS

2 cloves garlic

1 cup (240 g/8.5 oz) Ketchup (page 29)

2 tablespoons (30 ml/1 fl oz) apple cider vinegar

2 tablespoons (30 ml/1 fl oz) coconut aminos or fish sauce

2 tablespoons (10 g/0.4 oz) unsweetened cacao powder

2 tablespoons (20 g/0.7 oz) erythritol or Swerve

5 to 10 drops stevia

2 teaspoons paprika (regular or smoked)

1 teaspoon chile powder (mild or hot, to taste)

2 tablespoons (30 g/1.1 oz) butter or ghee

½ teaspoon smoked salt or regular sea salt

NUTRITION FACTS PER SERVING

(1 tablespoon/15 g)

Total carbs: 1.3 g

Fiber: 0.4 g

Net carbs: 0.9 g

Protein: 0.3 g

Fat: 1.1 g

Energy: 15 kcal

Macronutrient ratio:
Calories from carbs (24%), protein (8%), fat (68%)

Peel and crush the garlic. Place all the ingredients in a saucepan and cook over medium heat for 5 to 10 minutes. Transfer to a glass jar and keep in the fridge for up to a month.

TIP

Coconut aminos are a healthier alternative to soy sauce and are often recommended as a healthy soy sauce substitute on paleo diets. Soy products should be eaten in moderation, and some of them should be avoided completely. Unfortunately, most soy products come from genetically-modified (GMO) soybeans, and how GMO products affect health is still unclear. If you decide to use soy products, find ones that are made from non-GMO, fermented, unprocessed soy and that are gluten-free.

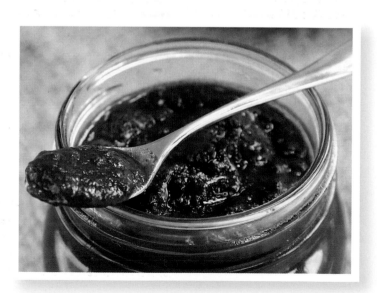

PESTO, THREE WAYS

Making your pesto at home is an easy way to add flavor and healthy fats to your diet, minus the additives that are often found in store-bought versions.

⅔ CUPS (160 G/5.6 OZ)	5 MINS	5 MINS

INGREDIENTS

½ cup (50 g/1.8 oz) pecans or walnuts, soaked for at least 1 hour

2 cups (30 g/1.1 oz) basil

2 cups (20 g/0.7 oz) arugula

4 cloves garlic

1 teaspoon fresh lemon zest

1 tablespoon (15 ml/0.5 fl oz) freshly squeezed lemon juice

¼ cup (60 ml/2 fl oz) extra virgin olive oil

Salt and freshly ground black pepper, to taste

Optional: ½ cup (45 g/1.6 oz) grated Parmesan cheese

NUTRITION FACTS PER SERVING

(2 tablespoons/30 g/1.1 oz)

Total carbs: 2.2 g

Fiber: 1 g

Net carbs: 1.2 g

Protein: 1.1 g

Fat: 15 g

Energy: 141 kcal

Macronutrient ratio: Calories from carbs (3%), protein (3%), fat (94%)

Drain the nuts and discard the water. Wash the basil and arugula. Place all the ingredients into a blender and pulse until smooth. Transfer to a jar and refrigerate. You can keep your pesto in the fridge for up to a week or two if it's stored properly: it helps to pour a thin layer of olive oil on the top, as it keeps it fresh for longer. Whenever you use the pesto, remember to add another thin layer of olive oil before you put it back in the fridge.

VARIATIONS

There are limitless varieties of pesto: simply combine your favorite herbs, nuts, seeds, herbs, and spices. (If you have a nut allergy, use sunflower seeds instead.) Try these variations:

Spinach Pesto: Place 2 cups (60 g/2.1 oz) spinach, ½ cup (65 g/2.3 oz) soaked macadamia nuts, (68 g/2.4 oz) pine nuts, or (75 g/2.7 oz) almonds, 4 cloves garlic, 2 spring onions, ¼ cup (60 ml/2 fl oz) olive oil, salt and freshly ground black pepper, to taste, and ½ cup (45 g/1.6 oz) Parmesan cheese (optional) into a blender and pulse until smooth.

Red Pesto: Place 1 cup (15 g/0.5 oz) basil, ½ cup (65 g/2.3 oz) soaked macadamia nuts, ½ cup (28 g/1 oz) sundried tomatoes, 2 tablespoons (30 g/1.1 oz) tomato puree, 1 tablespoon (15 ml/0.5 fl oz) freshly squeezed lemon juice, 2 cloves of garlic, and ½ cup (45 g/1.6 oz) Parmesan cheese (optional) into a blender and pulse until smooth.

TIP

If you can, use soaked and dehydrated nuts. If you want to preserve homemade pesto for longer, freeze it in manageable portions by spooning it into an ice cube tray. It'll keep in the freezer for up to 6 months. When you need it, just set the required amount in a bowl to thaw at room temperature until it melts.

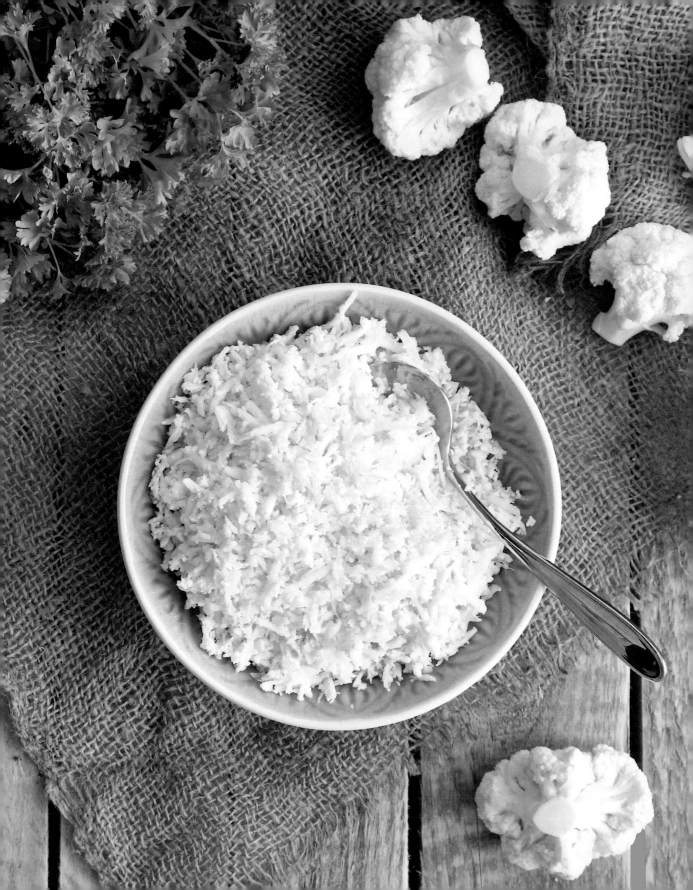

CAULI-RICE

Not only is cauliflower a perfect replacement for potatoes and rice, it's also ideal for thickening sauces without adding extra carbs and for making pizza bases. If you're following a healthy, low-carb diet, you should always have some Cauli-Rice on hand.

5 CUPS (600 G/21.2 OZ)	5 MINS	10 TO 15 MINS

INGREDIENTS
1 head cauliflower (600 g/ 21.2 oz)

NUTRITION FACTS
PER CUP (120 g/4.2 oz)

Total carbs: 6 g

Fiber: 2.4 g

Net carbs: 3.6 g

Protein: 2.3 g

Fat: 0.3 g

Energy: 30 kcal

Macronutrient ratio:
Calories from carbs (54%), protein (35%), fat (11%)

Remove the leaves and the hard core of the cauliflower and cut it into florets. Wash the cauliflower florets thoroughly and drain well. Once dry, run them through a hand grater or food processor with a regular blade or a grating blade; the latter will make the cauliflower look more like rice. Pulse until the florets resemble grains of rice. (Don't overdo it—it takes only a few more seconds to turn your Cauli-Rice into cauli-puree!) Refrigerate in an airtight container for up to four days. Cook your Cauli-Rice using these methods:

- **Steaming:** Place in a steam pot with boiling water and cook for 5 to 7 minutes.

- **Microwaving:** Transfer the processed cauliflower into a microwave-safe bowl and cook in the microwave on medium-high for 5 to 7 minutes. You won't need any water with this method.

- **Pan roasting:** Briefly cook the cauli-rice in a pan greased with butter or ghee or add it directly to the pot with whatever meat or sauce you plan to serve it with. This method adds extra flavor.

- **Baking:** Preheat the oven to 400°F (200°C, or gas mark 6). Spread the grated cauli-rice over a baking sheet lined with parchment paper and cook for 12 to 15 minutes, flipping two or three times. This method is useful when you want the cauli-rice to be as dry as possible.

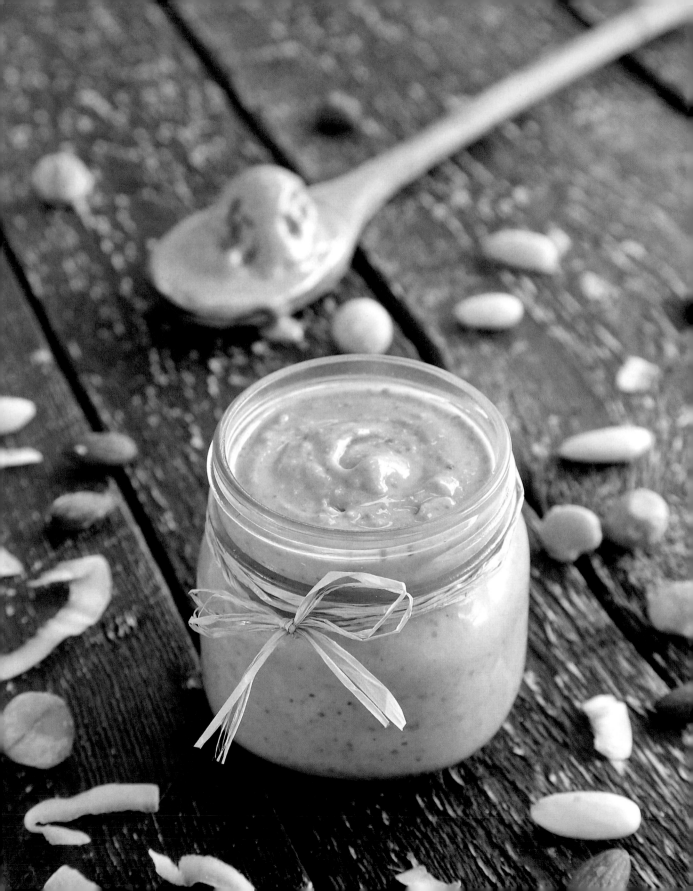

TOASTED NUT BUTTER

High in healthy monounsaturated fats, macadamia nuts are essential to the KetoDiet—and what's more, they're delicious in this easy-to-prepare nut butter.

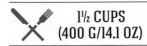 1½ CUPS (400 G/14.1 OZ)	10 MINS	25 TO 35 MINS

INGREDIENTS

1 cup (130 g/4.6 oz) macadamia nuts

1 cup (150 g/5.3 oz) almonds, blanched

2 cups (120 g/4.2 oz) desiccated coconut, flaked

NUTRITION FACTS PER SERVING

(2 tablespoons/32 g/1.1 oz)

Total carbs: 5.9 g

Fiber: 3.6 g

Net carbs: 2.3 g

Protein: 4 g

Fat: 20.2 g

Energy: 206 kcal

Macronutrient ratio: Calories from carbs (4%), protein (8%), fat (88%)

Preheat the oven to 350°F (175°C, or gas mark 4). Spread the nuts and flaked coconut evenly over a baking sheet and transfer to the oven. Bake for 12 to 15 minutes until slightly brown. Keep an eye on the nuts; if they burn, they will have an unpleasant bitter taste.

Remove from the oven and let cool for 10 minutes. Place the cooled nuts and coconut in a food processor and pulse until smooth and creamy. At first, the mixture will be dry. Scrape down the sides of your processor several times with a rubber spatula if the mixture sticks. This process may take up to 10 minutes depending on your processor.

Spoon the butter into a glass container and keep refrigerated or at room temperature. Try adding a tablespoon (15 g/0.5 oz) of it to a smoothie or use it to thicken sauces or make cookies (see Chocolate Chip & Orange Cookies, page 224).

SPICED BERRY JAM

Pair this sugar-free berry jam with full-fat yogurt, or use it as a secret weapon when you're creating luscious low-carb desserts. You can use any berries you like: either fresh or frozen will work just fine.

2 CUPS (640 G/22.6 OZ)	10 MINS	20 MINS

INGREDIENTS

1 cup (140 g/4.9 oz) strawberries

1 cup (125 g/4.4 oz) raspberries

1 cup (140 g/4.9 oz) blackberries

½ cup (75 g/2.6 oz) blueberries

½ teaspoon ground ginger or 1 teaspoon freshly grated ginger

½ teaspoon cinnamon

1 tablespoon (6 g/0.2 oz) orange zest

¼ teaspoon ground cloves

1 star anise, ground

2 tablespoons (20 g/0.7 oz) erythritol or Swerve

10 to 15 drops liquid stevia

2 tablespoons (16 g/0.5 oz) chia seeds

Wash the berries and place in a saucepan. Add all the remaining ingredients except for the chia seeds. Bring to a boil and then lower the heat. Cook for 5 to 8 minutes. Remove from the heat. Remove and discard the star anise.

Add the chia seeds and mix well. Let the jam sit for about 15 minutes before transferring to a lidded jar. Store in the fridge for up to two weeks.

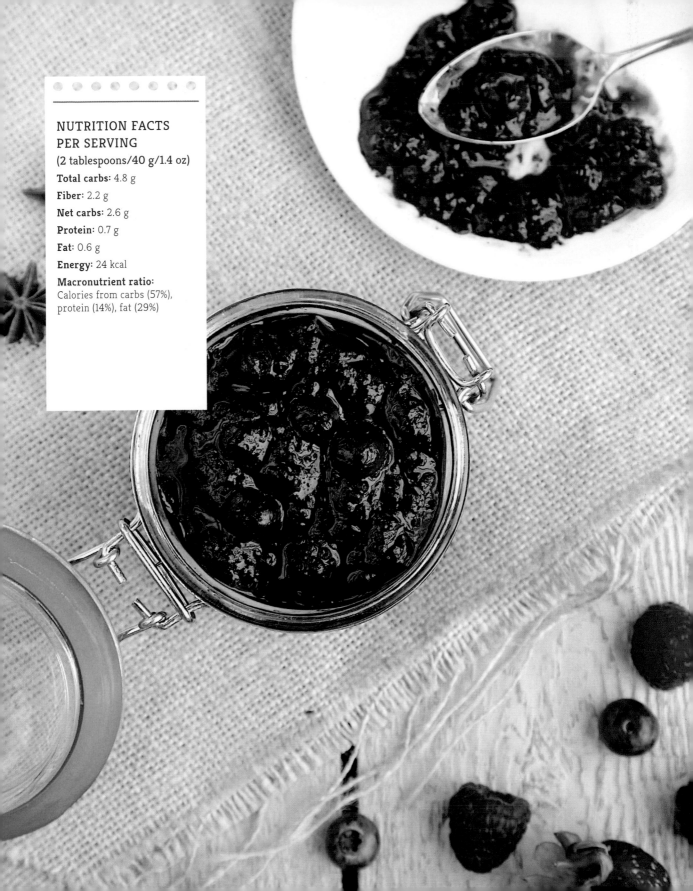

NUTRITION FACTS PER SERVING
(2 tablespoons/40 g/1.4 oz)

Total carbs: 4.8 g

Fiber: 2.2 g

Net carbs: 2.6 g

Protein: 0.7 g

Fat: 0.6 g

Energy: 24 kcal

Macronutrient ratio:
Calories from carbs (57%),
protein (14%), fat (29%)

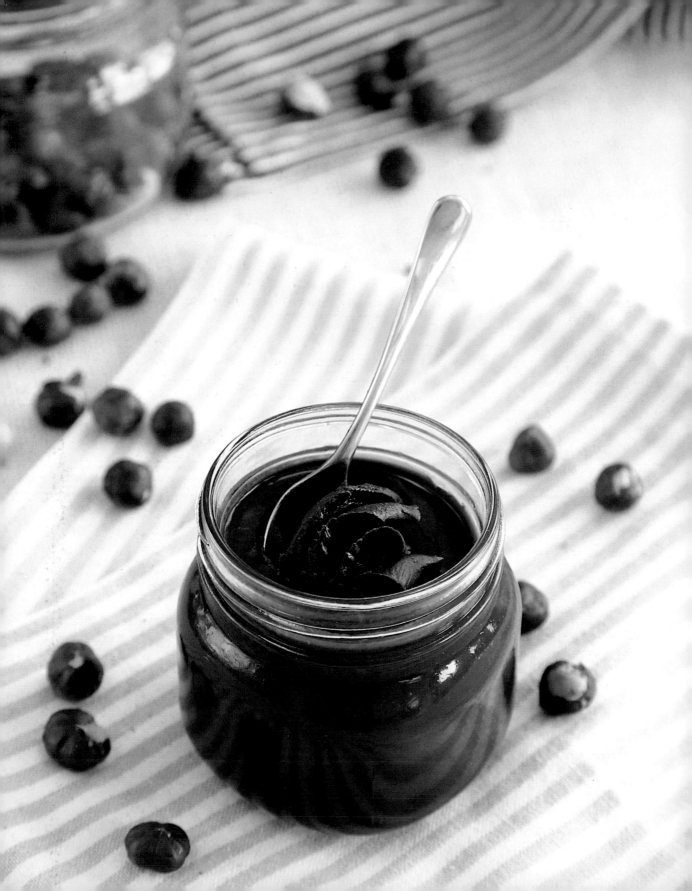

CHOCOLATE HAZELNUT BUTTER

If you love Nutella, you're in luck! This is a healthier version of the famous chocolate-hazelnut spread. It's high in heart-healthy monounsaturated fats, and it's sugar-free. Slather it on low-carb pancakes and waffles or use it in Chocolate Fat Bombs (see page 213).

2 CUPS (490 G/17.3 OZ)	5 MINS	25 TO 35 MINS

INGREDIENTS

1 cup (150 g/5.3 oz) hazelnuts

1 cup (130 g/4.6 oz) macadamia nuts

½ cup (75 g/2.6 oz) almonds

1 bar (100 g/3.5 oz) extra-dark chocolate, 85% cacao or more

1 tablespoon (15 g/0.5 oz) extra virgin coconut oil

1 vanilla bean or 1 teaspoon sugar-free vanilla extract

1 tablespoon (5 g/0.2 oz) cacao powder, unsweetened

2 tablespoons (20 g/0.7 oz) erythritol or Swerve, powdered

10 to 15 drops liquid stevia

Optional: ½ cup (120 ml/ 4 fl oz) coconut milk or heavy whipping cream

NUTRITION FACTS PER SERVING
(2 tablespoons/32 g/1.1 oz)

Total carbs: 5.9 g

Fiber: 2.9 g

Net carbs: 3 g

Protein: 3.9 g

Fat: 18.7 g

Energy: 193 kcal

Macronutrient ratio:
Calories from carbs (6%), protein (8%), fat (86%)

Preheat the oven to 375°F (190°C, or gas mark 5). Spread the hazelnuts, macadamia nuts, and almonds on a baking sheet and transfer to the oven. Bake for about 10 minutes until lightly browned.

Remove from the oven and let the nuts cool for 15 minutes. Meanwhile, melt the chocolate with the coconut oil in a water bath: Place a bowl over a pot with boiling water and let the chocolate melt, stirring frequently. Make sure the water doesn't touch the bottom of the bowl.

Rub the hazelnuts in your hands to remove the skins: this will help make the butter smooth and avoid the bitter taste imparted by the skins.

Place the nuts into a food processor and pulse until smooth. Cut the vanilla bean lengthwise and scrape out the seeds. Add the cacao powder, vanilla seeds, powdered erythritol, and liquid stevia to the melted chocolate. (To powder the erythritol, place it in a blender or coffee grinder and pulse until powdery for 15 to 20 seconds.) Pour the chocolate mixture into the nut mixture and pulse until smooth. If you're using the coconut milk, pour it into the hazelnut mixture and pulse again. Pour into a glass container and store in the fridge for up to 4 weeks.

Chapter Three:

BREAKFAST

When you give up grains and other high-carb foods, you might find yourself scratching your head over what to eat for breakfast. Without bread, pancakes, or cereals, is there even anything left? The answer is yes: real food that's packed with nutrients! Eggs, full-fat yogurt and cheese, nonstarchy vegetables, meats, nuts, and berries are all low-carb superfoods. This chapter is packed with easy-to-make breakfast meals that will keep you satiated until lunch: no snacking necessary. Brilliant keto-friendly breakfasts are just a few pages away!

KETO EGGS BENEDICT

Don't worry: you don't have to abandon your favorite brunch treats to go keto. Replace the English muffins in the traditional recipe with my Ultimate Keto Buns (see page 26) for an easy, low-carb take on this delicious classic.

1 SERVING	10 MINS	15 MINS

INGREDIENTS

1 serving Hollandaise Sauce (page 32)

Dash of red wine vinegar

Pinch of salt

1 large pastured egg

½ Ultimate Keto Bun (page 26)

2 slices (50 g/1.8 oz) pastured ham

1 tablespoon (2.5 g/0.08 oz) chopped fresh herbs (such as chives, parsley, or basil)

NUTRITION FACTS PER SERVING

Total carbs: 8.4 g

Fiber: 4.1 g

Net carbs: 4.3 g

Protein: 22.3 g

Fat: 43.5 g

Energy: 500 kcal

Macronutrient ratio: Calories from carbs (3%), protein (18%), fat (79%)

First, make the Hollandaise Sauce and keep it warm. To poach the egg, fill a small saucepan with water and then add the red wine vinegar and the salt. Bring to a boil over a medium-high heat.

Crack the egg into a cup. When the water is boiling, lower the cup into the water and gently slide the egg into the saucepan. Reduce the heat to low and cook for three minutes. (Use a timer to prevent overcooking.)

Remove the egg from the hot water with a slotted spoon and place it into a bowl of cold water for about a minute: this will prevent the egg from continuing to cook. Then remove the egg and drain it on a kitchen towel.

Set the halved Ultimate Keto Bun on a serving plate. Top with a slice of ham or two (if thin), followed by the poached egg, and then top with the Hollandaise Sauce. Finish with the chopped herbs.

BAKED SCOTCH EGGS

This is the ultimate comfort food! Make these Baked Scotch Eggs with homemade pork sausage meat and use pork rinds in place of breading. It's an extra low-carb meal that's great for either breakfast or lunch.

4 SERVINGS	20 MINS	45 MINS

INGREDIENTS

4 large pastured eggs

Sausage Meat

1 tablespoon (15 g/0.5 oz) ghee

1 package (100 g/3.5 oz) ham

0.9 pounds (400 g) ground pork, 20% fat

2 teaspoons paprika

1 teaspoon each dried sage and marjoram

¼ teaspoon ground cloves

½ teaspoon chile flakes

salt and black pepper to taste

"Breading"

½ cup (25 g/0.9 oz) ground pork rinds

2 tablespoons (14 g/0.5 oz) flax meal

Pinch salt and pepper

Optional: ½ cup (45 g/1.6 oz) grated Parmesan cheese

Preheat the oven to 350°F (175°C, or gas mark 4). First, hard boil the eggs.

Grease a pan with ghee and add the sliced ham. Cook over a medium-high heat for just about 3 minutes until lightly browned. (Alternatively, you can use bacon instead of ham: just omit the ghee.)

In a bowl, mix the ground pork with the browned ham, paprika, sage, marjoram, ground cloves, chili flakes, salt, and black pepper. Divide the meat into four parts, so you don't end up with spare eggs.

Flatten the meat and create hand-size burgers. Place the egg in the middle of the burger and wrap the meat around it. Make sure the egg is covered completely.

Mix the ground pork rinds with flax meal and season with salt and pepper. Add the Parmesan cheese if using. Roll the meat-wrapped eggs in the pork rind mixture until thoroughly coated.

Place the breaded meat on a baking sheet lined with parchment paper. Transfer to the oven and bake for about 25 minutes. Serve hot with mayonnaise, mustard, ketchup, or BBQ sauce.

NUTRITION FACTS PER SERVING

		Macronutrient ratio:
Total carbs: 2.8 g	**Protein:** 32.3 g	Calories from carbs
Fiber: 1.7 g	**Fat:** 33 g	(1%), protein (30%),
Net carbs: 1.1 g	**Energy:** 450 kcal	fat (69%)

EASTERN EUROPEAN HASH

Add super-healthy sauerkraut to your diet with this toothsome breakfast hash. Packed with celeriac and crowned with pastured sausages, it's best when it's topped with a fried egg or two.

 2 SERVINGS | **15 MINS** | **15 MINS**

INGREDIENTS

4 medium (260 g/9.2 oz) gluten-free sausages

1 medium (160 g/5.6 oz) celeriac

1 small (70 g/2.5 oz) white onion, peeled and chopped

1 cup (150 g/5.3 oz) sauerkraut

½ teaspoon caraway seeds

2 tablespoons (30 g/1.1 oz) ghee or butter

Salt and freshly ground black pepper, to taste

Optional: 2 large pastured eggs, fried

NUTRITION FACTS PER SERVING

Total carbs: 15.6 g

Fiber: 5.3 g

Net carbs: 10.3 g

Protein: 24.4 g

Fat: 38.4 g

Energy: 497 kcal

Macronutrient ratio:
Calories from carbs (9%), protein (20%), fat (71%)

Grease a pan with ghee and heat. Place the sausages in the hot pan and cook until browned. Turn two to three times to ensure the meat is evenly cooked. When done, remove the sausages from the pan and keep warm. Set the pan aside.

Peel and slice the celeriac with a julienne peeler or a vegetable spiralizer. If you don't have either, use the biggest holes on your box grater.

Put the onion in the pan you used for the sausages. Cook over medium-high heat for about 2 minutes, stirring frequently. Add the celeriac and cook for another 8 minutes; continue to stir frequently.

Add the sauerkraut and caraway seeds and combine well. Season with salt and black pepper. Heat the mixture through for about one minute until the sauerkraut is warm. Top with the sausages and fried eggs, if using.

ZUCCHINI & PUMPKIN HASH

*This easy, hearty, low-carb meal isn't just for breakfast:
it's fabulous at any time of the day.*

 2 SERVINGS | 10 MINS | 25 MINS

INGREDIENTS

1 tablespoon (15 g/0.5 oz) ghee, lard, or coconut oil

1 clove garlic, peeled and sliced

4 slices (60 g/2.1 oz) thinly-cut bacon, sliced

7.1 ounces (200 g) beef, ground

1 cup (120 g/4.2 oz) pumpkin, diced

½ teaspoon paprika

¼ teaspoon cinnamon

2 medium (400 g/14.1 oz) zucchini, diced

Salt and freshly ground black pepper, to taste

Optional: Fried pastured eggs or sliced avocado

NUTRITION FACTS PER SERVING

Total carbs: 11.2 g

Fiber: 2.7 g

Net carbs: 8.5 g

Protein: 24.5 g

Fat: 35.8 g

Energy: 460 kcal

Macronutrient ratio: Calories from carbs (7%), protein (22%), fat (71%)

Grease a pan with ghee and then throw in the garlic and cook over a medium heat for just a minute. Add the bacon and cook until crispy. Then add the ground beef and cook until browned.

Add the diced pumpkin and cook for 5 more minutes. Add paprika, cinnamon, and diced zucchini. Season with salt and black pepper to taste. Cook for another 10 to 15 minutes, stirring frequently. Remove from the heat and set aside. Serve immediately. Top with fried eggs or sliced avocado, if you wish.

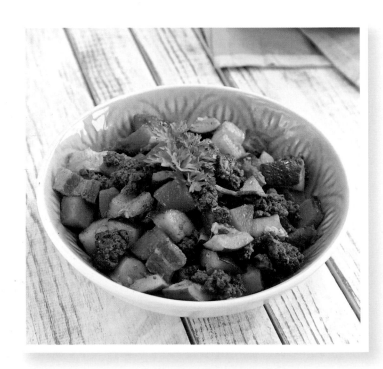

CHORIZO & KALE HASH

Leafy greens aren't just nutrient-dense; they're also very low in carbs, which means they're a KetoDiet staple. And they stand up so well to chorizo's lively flavor!

2 SERVINGS	10 MINS	25 MINS

INGREDIENTS

1 package (300 g/10.6 oz) dark-leaf kale

1 small (100 g/3.5 oz) rutabaga

2 tablespoons (30 g/1.1 oz) ghee

1 medium (60 g/2.1 oz) red onion, peeled and finely chopped

7.1 ounces (200 g) ground pork

2 ounces (56 g) Spanish chorizo or salami, sliced

Salt and freshly ground black pepper, to taste

Optional: Fried pastured eggs or sliced avocado

NUTRITION FACTS PER SERVING

Total carbs: 13.7 g

Fiber: 6.3 g

Net carbs: 7.4 g

Protein: 29.8 g

Fat: 49.6 g

Energy: 608 kcal

Macronutrient ratio: Calories from carbs (5%), protein (20%), fat (75%)

Wash and tear the kale into 2-inch (5 cm) pieces. Peel and dice the rutabaga or use a julienne peeler to create thin "noodles."

Grease a large pan with ghee and place on medium-high heat. When the pan is hot, toss in the onion. Cook for just about 3 minutes. When the onion is lightly browned, add the pork and cook for about 5 minutes, stirring frequently. Next, add the kale and rutabaga and cook for 10 to 15 minutes. Stir often to avoid burning.

Meanwhile, cook the chorizo in a separate pan until crispy. Add the chorizo and the juices to the pan with kale when done. Season with salt and black petter. Serve immediately.

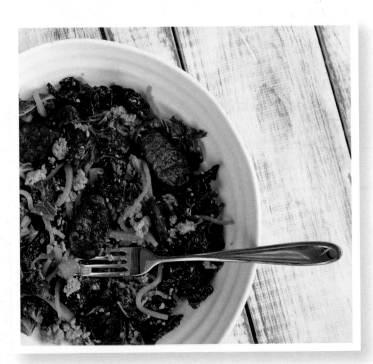

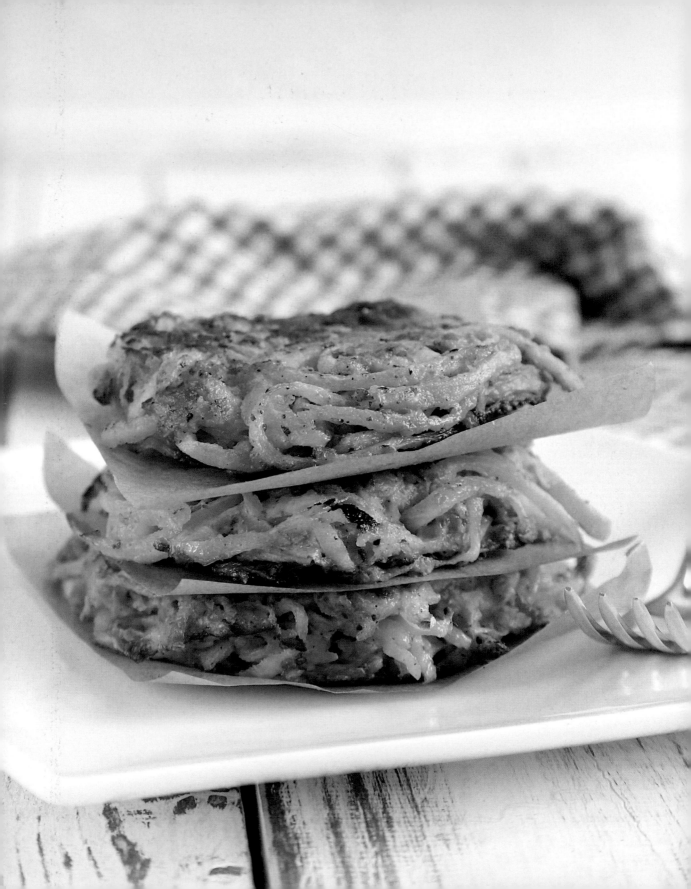

LOW-CARB LATKES

It might seem too good to be true, but it's not: you can make potato-free latkes! Serve these with sour cream, a fried egg, or a dollop of guacamole (see Ultimate GuacBurger on page 156).

 8 LATKES | **15 MINS** | **40 MINS**

INGREDIENTS

1 medium (400 g/14.1 oz) rutabaga

1 teaspoon salt

1 small (70 g/2.5 oz) white onion, peeled and sliced into small rings

1 large pastured egg

¼ cup (40 g/1.4 oz) flax meal

1 tablespoon (8 g/0.3 oz) psyllium husk powder

2 teaspoons dried marjoram

Freshly ground black pepper

4 tablespoons (60 g/2.1 oz) ghee, lard, or coconut oil

NUTRITION FACTS PER SERVING

(2 latkes)

Total carbs: 14.6 g

Fiber: 7.1 g

Net carbs: 7.5 g

Protein: 4.9 g

Fat: 20.7 g

Energy: 252 kcal

Macronutrient ratio:
Calories from carbs (13%), protein (8%), fat (79%)

Peel the rutabaga and then use a julienne peeler or a vegetable spiralizer to create thin rutabaga "noodles." Season with ½ teaspoon salt and let rest for 20 minutes.

Use a paper towel to pat the excess moisture off the rutabaga. Next, place both the rutabaga and onion into a mixing bowl and add the egg, flax meal, psyllium powder, and marjoram. Season with the remaining salt and pepper and mix until well combined.

Heat 2 tablespoons (30 g/1.1 oz) of ghee, lard, or coconut oil in a pan over a medium heat. Spoon the mixture into the pan to create two to four latkes at a time. Flatten each latke with the back of a spatula. Cook for 10 minutes on each side until golden brown.

Grease the pan with more ghee as needed and repeat with the remaining mixture. When done, serve immediately.

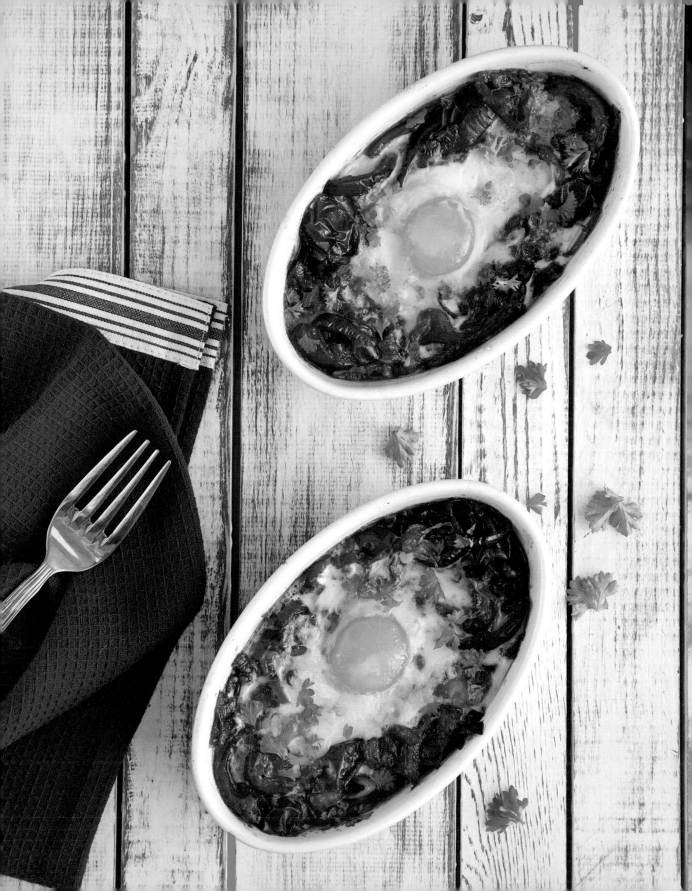

SPANISH EGGS

This spicy take on baked eggs is the best way to wake up lazy taste buds on a weekend morning. It's great on its own or with Ultimate Keto Buns (page 26).

 2 SERVINGS | **10 MINS** | **30 MINS**

INGREDIENTS

2 tablespoons (30 g/1.1 oz) ghee, lard, or coconut oil

½ small (30 g/2.1 oz) red onion, peeled and sliced

1 clove garlic, crushed

1 medium (120 g/4.2 oz) red pepper, seeded and sliced

1 small hot chile pepper

2 large pastured eggs

1 cup (240 g/8.5 oz) diced canned tomatoes

2 tablespoons (8 g/0.3 oz) chopped fresh parsley

Salt and freshly ground black pepper, to taste

Optional: ½ cup (56 g/2 oz) cheddar cheese, grated

NUTRITION FACTS PER SERVING

Total carbs: 10.9 g

Fiber: 2.9 g

Net carbs: 8.1 g

Protein: 8.3 g

Fat: 20.2 g

Energy: 257 kcal

Macronutrient ratio: Calories from carbs (13%), protein (13%), fat (74%)

Preheat the oven to 400°F (200°C, or gas mark 6). Grease a large pan with the ghee, lard, or coconut oil, and add the onion and garlic. Cook until translucent and then add the red pepper and chile pepper. Mix frequently and cook for about 10 minutes.

Stir in the tomatoes and parsley, saving some parsley for garnish. Cook for about a minute. Season with salt and black pepper and take off the heat. Spoon the mixture into two ovenproof dishes. Make a hollow in the middle of the mixture in each dish and crack an egg into each. Top the eggs with grated cheddar cheese, if you like. Bake in the oven for 15 to 20 minutes.

The eggs are done when the whites are cooked and the yolks are still runny. Remove from the oven, sprinkle with some more chopped parsley, and serve immediately.

BREAKFAST FRITTATA

*This easy, hearty, low-carb meal isn't just for breakfast:
it's fabulous at any time of the day.*

6 SERVINGS	10 MINS	40 TO 45 MINS

INGREDIENTS

10.6 ounces (300 g) ground beef

1 tablespoon (15 g/0.5 oz)
Dijon Mustard (page 31)

2 cloves garlic, crushed

1 teaspoon salt

2 tablespoons (30 g/1.1 oz)
ghee, lard, or coconut oil

1 large package spinach, fresh
(250 g/8.8 oz) or frozen
(275 g/9.7 oz)

10 large pastured eggs

2 tablespoons (4 g/0.14 oz)
chopped fresh parsley

1 teaspoon dried marjoram

Freshly ground black pepper

8.8 ounces (250 g) soft goat
cheese, crumbled

4 slices (60 g/2.1 oz) thinly-cut
bacon, chopped

NUTRITION FACTS
PER SERVING

Total carbs: 3.4 g

Fiber: 1.4 g

Net carbs: 2 g

Protein: 29.9 g

Fat: 34.8 g

Energy: 450 kcal

Macronutrient ratio:
Calories from carbs (2%),
protein (27%), fat (71%)

Preheat the oven to 400°F (200°C, or gas mark 6). In a bowl, combine the beef, Dijon mustard, crushed garlic, and half of the salt. Mix well. Form the mixture into small meatballs and set aside.

Wash and dry the spinach if using fresh. Grease a large pan with ghee, lard, or coconut oil and add the spinach. Cook until wilted and remove from the heat.

Crack the eggs into a large bowl and whisk with a fork. Add the herbs and season with salt and black pepper. Pour the eggs into a large caserole dish.

Add the spinach, crumbled goat cheese, and raw meatballs to the eggs. Finish with the sliced bacon. Bake for 40 to 45 minutes. Let the frittata stand for a few minutes before serving.

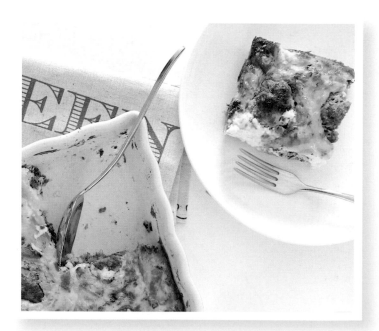

SPINACH & FETA CREPES

This recipe takes its inspiration from Greek cuisine, and it's both healthy and filling: one crepe is great as a starter, and two are enough to keep you going until lunch.

 2 SERVINGS | **10 MINS** | **15 MINS**

INGREDIENTS

2 servings (4 medium-sized) Essential Keto Crepes (page 24)

1 medium package spinach, fresh (150 g/5.3 oz) or frozen (160 g/5.6 oz)

2 tablespoons (30 g/1.1 oz) ghee, lard, or coconut oil

1 clove garlic, crushed

1 tablespoon (8 g/0.3 oz) chopped fresh parsley

1 tablespoon (6 g/0.2 oz) chopped fresh mint

Optional: pinch ground sumac

Freshly ground black pepper, to taste

1 large pastured egg

1 cup (150 g/5.3 oz) crumbled feta cheese

Salt, to taste

NUTRITION FACTS PER SERVING

Total carbs: 12.4 g

Fiber: 4.5 g

Net carbs: 7.9 g

Protein: 26.4 g

Fat: 53.1 g

Energy: 630 kcal

Macronutrient ratio: Calories from carbs (5%), protein (17%), fat (78%)

Prepare the crepes. Wash and dry the spinach if using fresh. Grease a large pan with ghee, lard, or coconut oil. When hot, add the crushed garlic and cook for a minute. Toss in the spinach and cook until wilted or thawed. Add the chopped herbs, the black pepper, and the sumac, if using.

Crack in the egg and cook for another 2 to 3 minutes, stirring frequently. Add the feta cheese and cook for another minute while stirring. Take off the heat and season with salt if needed.

Place a quarter of the filling on each crepe. Fold each crepe in half twice and serve immediately. For a dairy-free alternative to feta cheese, try Simple Shredded Chicken (page 128).

EGG MUFFIN IN A CUP

What's the speediest way to whip up a healthy breakfast?
The answer is simple: these one-minute egg muffins!

1 SERVING	5 MINS	5 MINS

INGREDIENTS

⅓ cup (56 g/2 oz) chopped vegetables, such as broccoli, asparagus, or spinach

1 tablespoon (15 g/0.5 oz) ghee or butter

1 tablespoon (6 g/0.2 oz) sun-dried tomatoes, drained and chopped

3 tablespoons (15 g/0.5 oz) grated Parmesan cheese, or a slice of crispy bacon

1 large pastured egg

Pinch salt and pepper

NUTRITION FACTS PER SERVING

Total carbs: 5.1 g

Fiber: 1.7 g

Net carbs: 3.4 g

Protein: 13.4 g

Fat: 24.6 g

Energy: 294 kcal

Macronutrient ratio: Calories from carbs (5%), protein (18%), fat (77%)

Place all the vegetables except the spinach, if you're using it, into a large mug with 1 tablespoon (15 g/0.5 oz) of ghee. Cook them in the microwave for 1 minute if the vegetables are precooked or for 2 to 3 minutes for raw vegetables.

Add the spinach and cheese or crispy bacon and crack in the egg. Season with salt and black pepper, and put the mug back into the microwave for another minute.

TIP

You can easily make this quick meal at work: Just store all the ingredients in an airtight container and then place in a mug, crack in the egg, and cook in a microwave.

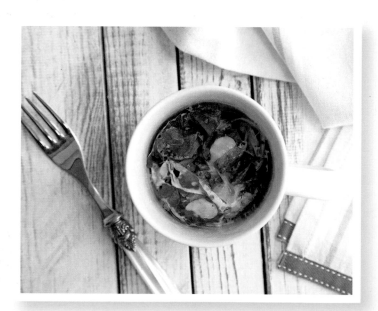

VANILLA PROTEIN WAFFLES

Who doesn't love waffles? And they're so easy to prepare.
Make a batch in advance and store them in the freezer: that
way, you'll always have a healthy breakfast on hand.

4 WAFFLES	10 MINS	15 MINS

INGREDIENTS

¼ cup (30 g/1.1 oz) coconut flour

¼ cup (25 g/0.9 oz) whey protein powder or pastured egg white protein powder, vanilla or unflavored

¼ teaspoon baking soda

½ teaspoon cream of tartar

1 tablespoon (10 g/0.4 oz) erythritol or Swerve

2 large pastured eggs

½ cup (120 ml/4 fl oz) almond milk

2 tablespoons (30 ml/1 fl oz) melted extra virgin coconut oil

1 vanilla bean or 1 teaspoon sugar-free vanilla extract

10 to 15 drops stevia

Optional: 4 tablespoons (80 g/ 2.8 oz) Spiced Berry Jam (page 40) or 2 tablespoons (30 g/1.1 oz) butter

Sift the coconut flour to avoid any lumps. Place all the dry ingredients in a bowl and mix well. Set aside.

In another bowl, crack in the eggs and add the almond milk, melted coconut oil, vanilla, and liquid stevia and whisk well. Add the dry ingredients to the egg mixture and combine well.

Pour the batter into a waffle maker and then close and cook for a minute or two (the exact time depends on the waffle maker). Serve with butter or Spiced Berry Jam.

Store any leftover waffles in an airtight container in the fridge for up to five days or freeze for longer.

TIP

When it comes to protein powders, I recommend whey protein isolate: it has no artificial sweeteners or colorings, and it's GMO- and hormone-free. If you prefer one with sweeteners, get one with no aspartame or artificial additives. Just remember: The amount of total carbohydrates per 100 g should be no more than 6 g. Instead of whey protein, you can also use egg white powder or gelatin powder from grass-fed cows.

NUTRITION FACTS PER SERVING (2 waffles)

Total carbs: 7.2 g

Fiber: 3.8 g

Net carbs: 3.4 g

Protein: 19 g

Fat: 20.7 g

Energy: 294 kcal

Macronutrient ratio: Calories from carbs (5%), protein (27%), fat (68%)

CRISPY BACON PANCAKES

This is a delicious, sweet-and-salty, keto-friendly breakfast that's perfect for long Sunday mornings.

8 PANCAKES	15 MINS	30 MINS

INGREDIENTS

Pancakes

8 slices (120 g/4.2 oz) of thinly-cut bacon

¼ cup (30 g/1.1 oz) coconut flour

¾ cup (75 g/2.6 oz) almond flour

¼ cup (25 g/0.9 oz) whey protein or pastured egg white protein, vanilla or unflavored

¼ cup (40 g/1.4 oz) erythritol or Swerve, powdered

½ teaspoon baking soda

1 teaspoon cream of tartar

4 large pastured eggs

¼ cup (55 g/1.9 oz) coconut oil, ghee or butter, melted plus more for frying

½ cup (120 ml/4 fl oz) almond milk (or ¼ cup [60 ml/2 fl oz] coconut milk plus ¼ cup [60 ml/2 fl oz] water)

10 to 15 drops liquid stevia

Chocolate dip

2 tablespoons (10 g/0.4 oz) cacao powder, unsweetened

¼ cup (55 g/1.9 oz) extra virgin coconut oil

2 tablespoons (20 g/0.7 oz) erythritol or Swerve, powdered

First, prepare the crispy bacon. Preheat the oven to 375°F (190°C, or gas mark 5). Line a baking sheet with parchment paper. Lay the bacon strips out flat on the paper, leaving space so they don't overlap. Place the tray in the oven and cook for about 10 to 15 minutes until the bacon is browned. Remove the tray from the oven and transfer the bacon to a serving plate.

For the pancakes, first combine the coconut flour, almond flour, whey protein powder, erythritol, baking soda, and cream of tartar into a bowl and mix well.

Crack the eggs in a separate bowl and add the melted coconut oil, almond milk, and liquid stevia. Slowly add the dry ingredients to the wet and keep mixing until well combined.

Heat a large pan greased with coconut oil. When hot, pour in the batter: you can use a piping bag for precise shapes or a regular spoon for oval pancakes.

As the pancakes are cooking, top each one with a slice of crispy bacon and cook until small bubbles start to appear along the edges of each pancake. Then flip to the other side and cook for another minute.

For the chocolate dip, mix the cacao powder, melted coconut oil, and erythritol and serve with the pancakes.

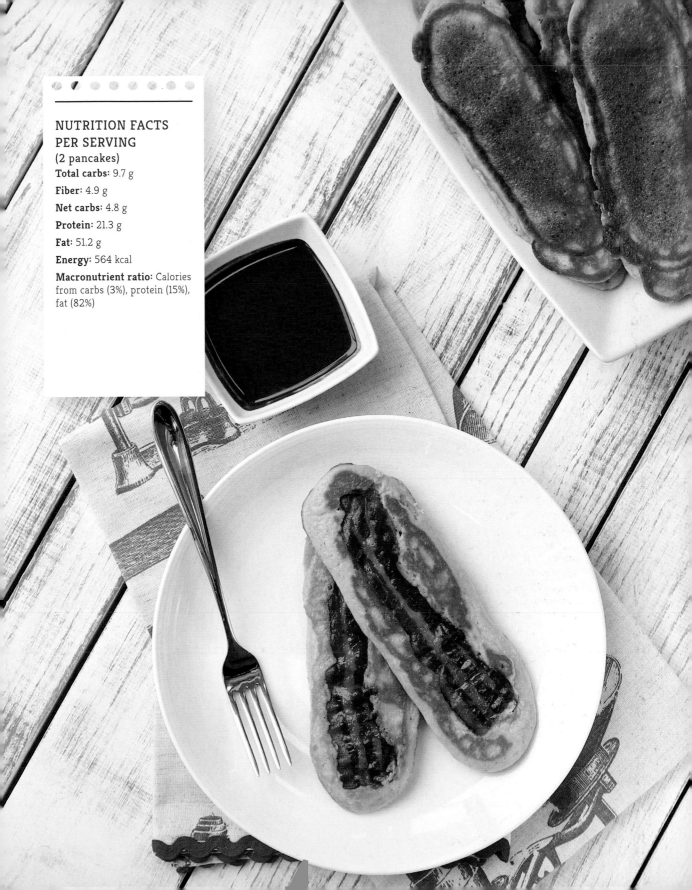

NUTRITION FACTS
PER SERVING
(2 pancakes)

Total carbs: 9.7 g

Fiber: 4.9 g

Net carbs: 4.8 g

Protein: 21.3 g

Fat: 51.2 g

Energy: 564 kcal

Macronutrient ratio: Calories from carbs (3%), protein (15%), fat (82%)

VANILLA & BERRY CHIA PARFAIT

Chia seeds are high in fiber and minerals and low in net carbs, which means they're great for inducing satiety and promoting healthy weight loss. There's finally a healthy way to enjoy dessert for breakfast!

2 SERVINGS	5 MINS	5 MINS + CHILLING

INGREDIENTS

1 vanilla bean (or 1 teaspoon sugar-free vanilla extract)

¼ cup (30 g/1.1 oz) chia seeds

¾ cup (180 ml/6 fl oz) almond milk

¼ cup (60 ml/2 fl oz) coconut milk

5 to 10 drops liquid stevia

Optional: 2 tablespoons (20 g/0.7 oz) erythritol or Swerve, powdered

⅓ cup (70 g/2.5 oz) Spiced Berry Jam (page 40)

½ cup (115 g/4.1 oz) sour cream or creamed coconut milk

NUTRITION FACTS PER SERVING

Total carbs: 13.9 g

Fiber: 7.9 g

Net carbs: 6 g

Protein: 5.8 g

Fat: 23.8 g

Energy: 279 kcal

Macronutrient ratio: Calories from carbs (9%), protein (9%), fat (82%)

Cut the vanilla bean lengthwise and scrape out the seeds. Mix the vanilla seeds, chia seeds, almond milk, and coconut milk. (If you prefer a smooth texture, use ground chia seeds instead of whole.) Sweeten with liquid stevia to taste and add the erythritol, if using. Let the mixture sit in the fridge for at least 15 minutes or overnight.

Then, start layering the parfait. Divide half of the chia seed "pudding" between two glass jars and reserve the other half for later. Add a layer of Spiced Berry Jam, then a layer of sour cream, and repeat until all the ingredients have been used. Serve immediately or keep in the fridge for up to three days.

HOW TO CREAM COCONUT MILK

Instead of sour cream, you can use creamed coconut milk. To cream coconut milk, simply place the can in the fridge overnight. Then, open the can and spoon out the solidified coconut milk. Discard the liquids. Do not shake the can before opening.

PUMPKIN MUG CAKE

Fresh, hot, low-carb pumpkin muffins that are ready in just two minutes? Yes, please!

 1 SERVING | **5 MINS** | **5 MINS**

Place all the ingredients in a microwave-safe mug and mix with a spoon. Microwave on high for about 2 minutes. Serve with full-fat yogurt, sour cream, or creamed coconut milk.

INGREDIENTS

2 tablespoons (40 g/1.4 oz) pumpkin puree

1 tablespoon (12 g/0.4 oz) coconut flour

2 tablespoons (16 g/0.6 oz) almond flour

1 tablespoon (8 g/0.3 oz) chia seeds, ground

1 large pastured egg

1 tablespoon (15 g/0.5 oz) coconut oil, ghee, or butter

2 tablespoons (20 g/0.8 oz) erythritol or Swerve

½ teaspoon pumpkin-spice mix (cinnamon, nutmeg, ginger, cloves and allspice)

⅛ teaspoon baking soda

Optional: 5 to 10 drops liquid stevia

Optional: a dollop of full-fat yogurt, whipped cream, sour cream, or coconut milk

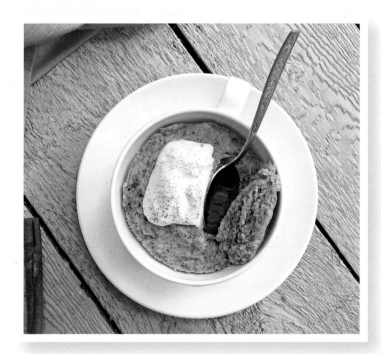

NUTRITION FACTS PER SERVING

Total carbs: 14.6 g	**Protein:** 13.9 g	**Macronutrient ratio:** Calories from carbs (7%), protein (15%), fat (78%)
Fiber: 8.2 g	**Fat:** 31.3 g	
Net carbs: 6.3 g	**Energy:** 385 kcal	

CHOCOLATE & ORANGE SPICED GRANOLA

Grain-free granola is easy to prepare, and it's perfect for breakfast, a healthy dessert, or a quick snack.

10 SERVINGS	5 MINS	1 HOUR

INGREDIENTS

Dry Ingredients
1 cup (140 g/5 oz) almonds

1 cup (100 g/3.5 oz) pecans

1 cup (75 g/2.6 oz) shredded desiccated coconut

1 cup (60 g/2.1 oz) flaked desiccated coconut

½ cup (50 g/1.8 oz) almond flour

¼ cup (30 g/1.1 oz) chia seeds

¼ cup (30 g/1.1 oz) pumpkin seeds

½ cup (50 g/1.8 oz) whey protein or pastured egg white protein powder, chocolate or unflavored

½ cup (80 g/2.8 oz) erythritol or Swerve

¼ cup (20 g/0.7 oz) cacao powder, unsweetened

2 tablespoons (12 g/0.4 oz) fresh organic orange zest (or 1 tablespoon/6 g/0.2 oz dried)

1 tablespoon (7 g/0.25 oz) cinnamon

½ teaspoon salt

Wet Ingredients
1 large pastured egg white

¼ cup (56 g/2 oz) butter, ghee or coconut oil, melted

15 to 20 drops liquid stevia

2 tablespoons (30 ml/1 fl oz) water

Preheat the oven to 300°F (150°C, or gas mark 2). Roughly chop the almonds and pecans. Place all the dry ingredients—the almonds through the salt—in a mixing bowl and combine well.

Add the egg white, melted butter, ghee, or oil, liquid stevia, and water. Mix well until the mixture resembles crumbly dough.

Transfer the mixture to a baking sheet lined with parchment paper. Bake for 30 to 40 minutes, turning halfway through the cooking process. Remove from the oven and let the granola cool.

When it's reached room temperature, transfer the granola to a glass container and have it for breakfast! Serve it with coconut milk, almond milk, cream, full-fat yogurt, or sour cream.

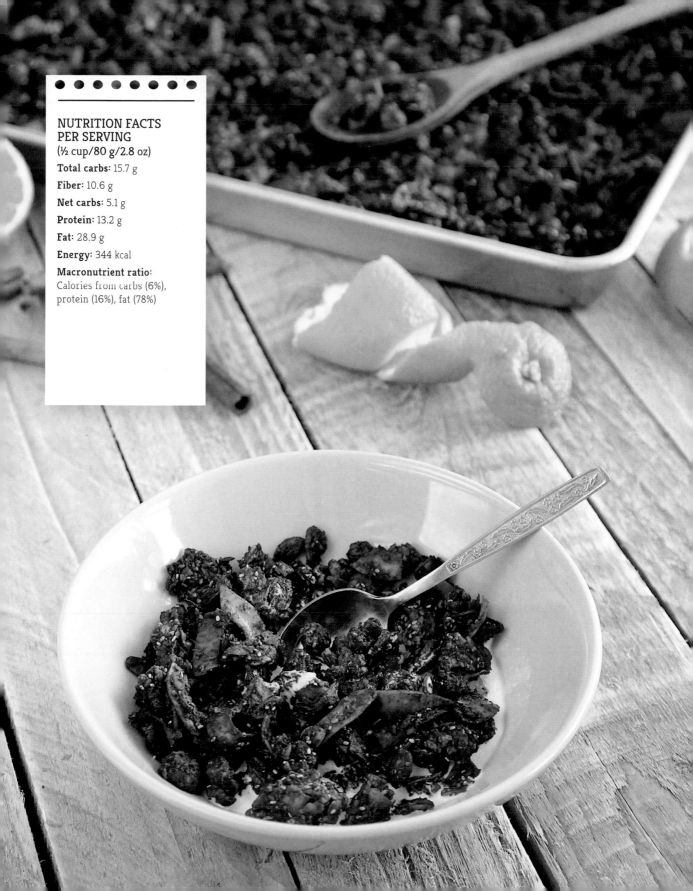

**NUTRITION FACTS
PER SERVING**
(½ cup/80 g/2.8 oz)

Total carbs: 15.7 g

Fiber: 10.6 g

Net carbs: 5.1 g

Protein: 13.2 g

Fat: 28.9 g

Energy: 344 kcal

Macronutrient ratio:
Calories from carbs (6%),
protein (16%), fat (78%)

SWEET CINNAMON ROLLS

Grab one of these fluffy, sweet cinnamon rolls for a quick breakfast or for a satisfying dessert: they're high in fiber and will keep hunger at bay.

 10 ROLLS | 20 MINS | 1 HOUR

INGREDIENTS

Dough

2 cups (200 g/7.1 oz) almond flour

⅓ cup (40 g/1.4 oz) coconut flour

¼ cup (25 g/0.9 oz) whey protein or egg white protein powder, vanilla or unflavored or more almond flour

⅔ cup (80 g/2.8 oz) psyllium husk powder

½ cup (80 g/2.8 oz) erythritol or Swerve, powdered

15 to 20 drops liquid stevia

¼ teaspoon salt

1 teaspoon baking soda

2 teaspoons cream of tartar

2 large pastured eggs

6 large pastured egg whites

1¼ cup (300 ml/10.1 fl oz) hot water

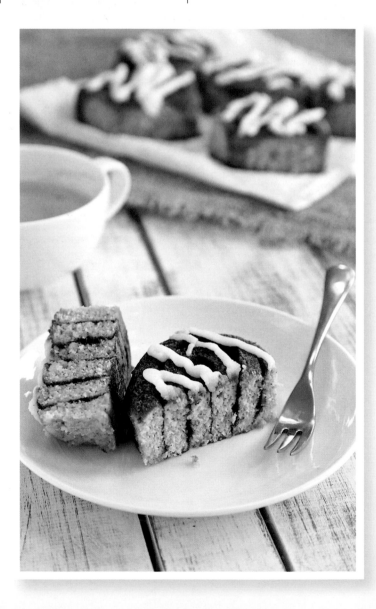

Filling

2 tablespoons (30 g/1.1 oz) coconut oil, ghee, or butter, softened but not melted

1 tablespoon (8 g) cinnamon

¼ cup (40 g/1.4 oz) erythritol or Swerve

Pinch salt

Icing

⅓ cup (80 g/2.8 oz) coconut butter, melted

1 tablespoon (15 g/0.5 oz) extra virgin coconut oil, melted

Optional: 10 to 15 drops liquid stevia or 2 tablespoons (20 g/0.7 oz) erythritol or Swerve, powedered

NUTRITION FACTS PER ROLL

Total carbs: 14.7 g

Fiber: 10.4 g

Net carbs: 4.4 g

Protein: 7.7 g

Fat: 19.6 g

Energy: 230 kcal

Macronutrient ratio:
Calories from carbs (8%), protein (14%), fat (78%)

Preheat the oven to 325°F (165°C, or gas mark 3). To make the dough, place the almond flour,coconut flour, protein powder, and psyllium husk powder into a mixer. (Note: Don't use whole psyllium husks; run them through a blender or a coffee grinder if necessary.) Add powdered erythritol, salt, baking soda, and cream of tartar and mix until well combined. Add the eggs and egg whites and process well. Pour in the hot water and process until well combined.

Lay out a sheet of parchment paper or foil on a flat work surface. Transfer the dough to the parchment paper and flatten with your hands. Place the dough on parchment paper on a flat work surface and set another piece of parchment or foil on top. Roll the dough out until thin, about ½-inch-thick (1.3 cm) rectangular shape. The sides should be about 14 inches (36 cm) long.Meanwhile, prepare the filling. Mix the softened coconut oil, cinnamon, erythritol, and salt until creamy.

Spread the cinnamon filling over the dough, leaving a ½- to 1-inch (1.3 to 2.5 cm) space along each side. Roll up the dough and cut it in half. Then cut each half into 5 pieces to create 10 equal servings.

Place all the rolls cut-side down on a large baking tray except the first and last slices: set these cut-side up. Transfer the tray to the oven and bake for about 40 minutes. When done, remove the tray from the oven and leave the cinnamon rolls to cool.

Prepare the icing by mixing the melted coconut butter with coconut oil. Optionally, add stevia or erythritol and mix well. Drizzle the coconut butter mixture over the cooled rolls. Store in a cool place for up to three days or in the fridge for up to a week.

TIP

Don't waste the egg yolks! Keep them for other recipes, like Lamb Avgolemono (page 180), Keto Crème Brûlée (page 214), Mayonnaise (page 28), or Hollandaise Sauce (page 32).

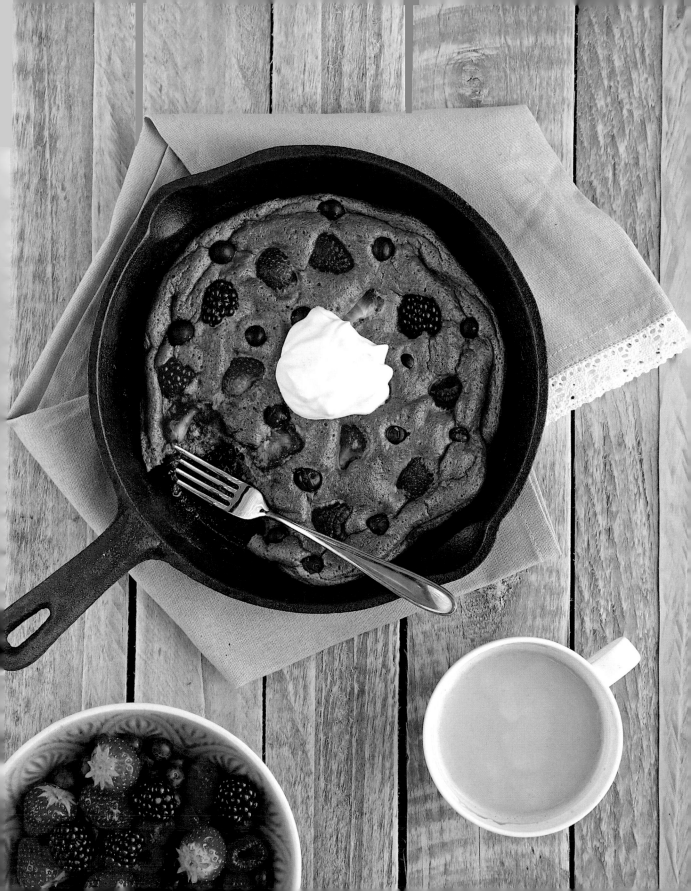

FLUFFY COCOA & BERRY OMELET

A sweet omelet that's as light as a chocolate cloud, my Fluffy Cocoa & Berry Omelet makes a great weekend breakfast treat.

1 SERVING	10 MINS	15 MINS

INGREDIENTS

2 tablespoons (20 g/0.7 oz) erythritol or Swerve, powdered

Optional: 5 to 10 drops liquid stevia, for a sweeter taste

3 large pastured eggs

1 tablespoon (5 g/0.2 oz) cacao powder

¼ teaspoon cream of tartar

1 tablespoon (15 g/0.5 oz) ghee or coconut oil

⅓ cup (50 g/1.8 oz) mixed berries (strawberries, raspberries, blueberries or blackberries)

Optional: Dollop of whipped cream, sour cream, or creamed coconut milk

NUTRITION FACTS PER SERVING

Total carbs: 10 g

Fiber: 2.8 g

Net carbs: 7.2 g

Protein: 20.3 g

Fat: 30 g

Energy: 383 kcal

Macronutrient ratio:
Calories from carbs (8%), protein (21%), fat (71%)

Set the oven to broil at 500°F (260°C, or gas mark 10). To ensure that the omelet has a smooth texture, place the erythritol into a blender and pulse until powdered.

Separate the egg whites from the yolks. Put the egg yolks into a bowl and set aside. Using an electric mixer or a hand whisk, start whisking the egg whites and add the cream of tartar as you go. Add in the erythritol, liquid stevia (if using), and cacao powder and beat until the egg whites create soft peaks.

In another bowl, mix the egg yolks with a fork and then gently fold in the egg whites. Mix gently so you don't deflate the egg mixture.

Meanwhile, wash the berries and pat them dry. Grease a hot ovenproof pan with ghee, fold in the omelet mixture, and then sprinkle with the berries. Cook on low heat for about 5 minutes until the bottom of the omelet starts to brown. At that point, remove from the stovetop and place in the oven under the broiler for about 5 minutes.

When done, the top should be slightly brown and crispy while the inside is still soft. Optionally, top with whipped cream, sour cream, or creamed coconut milk.

HOT KETO PORRIDGE

The healthy fats and protein in this sugar- and grain-free porridge will help you stay fuller for longer.

 2 SERVINGS | 5 MINS | 10 MINS

Combine all the ingredients in a saucepan and mix until well combined. Cook for about 3 to 5 minutes, stirring, until the egg is cooked. Add a few drops of liquid stevia or serve with extra dark chocolate or berries, if you like.

INGREDIENTS

¼ cup (65 g/2.3 oz) Toasted Nut Butter (page 39)

2 tablespoons (12 g/0.4 oz) shredded desiccated coconut

2 tablespoons (20 g/0.7 oz) pecan nuts, roughly chopped

2 tablespoons (16 g/0.5 oz) chia seeds

2 tablespoons (30 ml/1 fl oz) coconut milk or heavy whipping cream

¼ cup (60 ml/2 fl oz) almond milk

1 large pastured egg

½ teaspoon cinnamon

Optional: 5 to 10 drops stevia, 1 ounce dark chocolate or ¼ cup berries

NUTRITION FACTS PER SERVING

Total carbs: 13.1 g

Fiber: 8.7 g

Net carbs: 4.5 g

Protein: 11.3 g

Fat: 36.8 g

Energy: 408 kcal

Macronutrient ratio: Calories from carbs (4%), protein (12%), fat (84%)

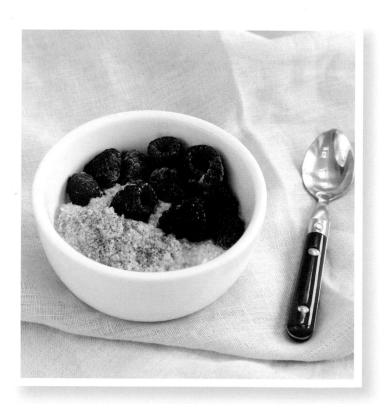

Chapter Four:

SAVORY SNACKS

Sometimes, life gets in the way, and you just don't have time to cook a full keto-friendly meal when you'd like to. So be sure to have a supply of these savory snacks on hand: that way, you won't be tempted to resort to sugary or carb-laden convenience foods. Simple to make, portable, high in healthy fats, and low in carbs, the recipes in this chapter are here to help. They're exactly what you need if you've got a busy day ahead of you at the office or if you need a little something to keep you going until dinnertime.

SAVORY FAT BOMBS

This is a savory alternative to the popular fat bombs— and they're great for a fat fast!

6 TRUFFLES	10 MINS	1 HOUR

INGREDIENTS

3.5 oz (100 g) cream cheese

¼ cup (55 g/1.9 oz) butter

2 large (60 g/2.1 oz) slices of bacon

1 medium (15 g/0.5 oz) spring onion or chives

1 clove garlic, crushed

Salt and freshly ground black pepper, to taste

NUTRITION FACTS PER TRUFFLE

Total carbs: 0.6 g

Fiber: 0.1 g

Net carbs: 0.5 g

Protein: 2.1 g

Fat: 11.7 g

Energy: 108 kcal

Macronutrient ratio: Calories from carbs (2%), protein (7%), fat (91%)

Place the cream cheese into a bowl. Cut the butter into smaller pieces and add to the cream cheese. Leave at room temperature to soften.

Meanwhile, prepare the bacon. Crisp up the bacon on both sides in hot pan and set aside. Let the bacon cool slightly before breaking it up into small pieces.

Chop the spring onion and soak in a bowl of water for one minute: all the dirt will settle at the bottom of the bowl. Remove the chopped onion and drain well on a paper towel.

Add the garlic to the room-temperature cream cheese and butter. Mix well using an electric beater or a hand whisk.

Add the bacon grease and bacon pieces. Set some bacon aside for topping. Season with salt and black pepper and mix well.

Line a clean tray with parchment paper and use a spoon to create small mounds of the mixture (about 2 tablespoons/ 30 g/1.1 oz each). Place in the fridge for 30 to 60 minutes to set. Alternatively, simply transfer the mixture to an airtight container and refrigerate: when ready to serve, just spoon out 2 tablespoons (30 g/1.1 oz) per serving. Store in the fridge for up to 3 days.

KETO HUMMUS

Traditional hummus, which is made from chickpeas, is high in carbs. This version is both low-carb and paleo-friendly!

4 SERVINGS	5 MINS	10 TO 15 MINS

INGREDIENTS

5.3 ounces (150 g) macadamia nuts

Optional: Handful (30 g/1.1 oz) cashew nuts

3 cloves garlic, peeled

¼ cup (60 g/2.1 oz) tahini

¼ cup (60 ml/2 fl oz) extra virgin olive oil

2 to 4 tablespoons (30 to 60 ml) lemon or lime juice

¼ cup (60 ml/2 fl oz) water

2 tablespoons (4 g/0.1 oz) chopped fresh tarragon (or basil or parsley)

½ teaspoon salt

Freshly ground black pepper

NUTRITION FACTS PER SERVING

Total carbs: 10.3 g

Fiber: 4.8 g

Net carbs: 5.5 g

Protein: 5.8 g

Fat: 50.5 g

Energy: 490 kcal

Macronutrient ratio:
Calories from carbs (4%), protein (5%), fat (91%)

Preheat the oven to 350°F (175°C, or gas mark 5). Place the macadamia nuts (and cashews, if using) on a baking sheet and roast in the oven for about 10 minutes, stirring once or twice to prevent burning.

Mash the peeled garlic before blending to avoid leaving large pieces in the sauce.

Place the roasted nuts, garlic, and tahini in a blender. Add extra virgin olive oil, lime or lemon juice, and water. Blend until smooth and transfer to a bowl.

Add the chopped herbs. Season with salt and black pepper and mix well. Serve with freshly-cut vegetables such as cucumbers, celery stalks, or bell peppers.

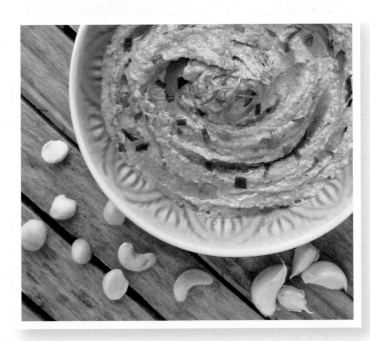

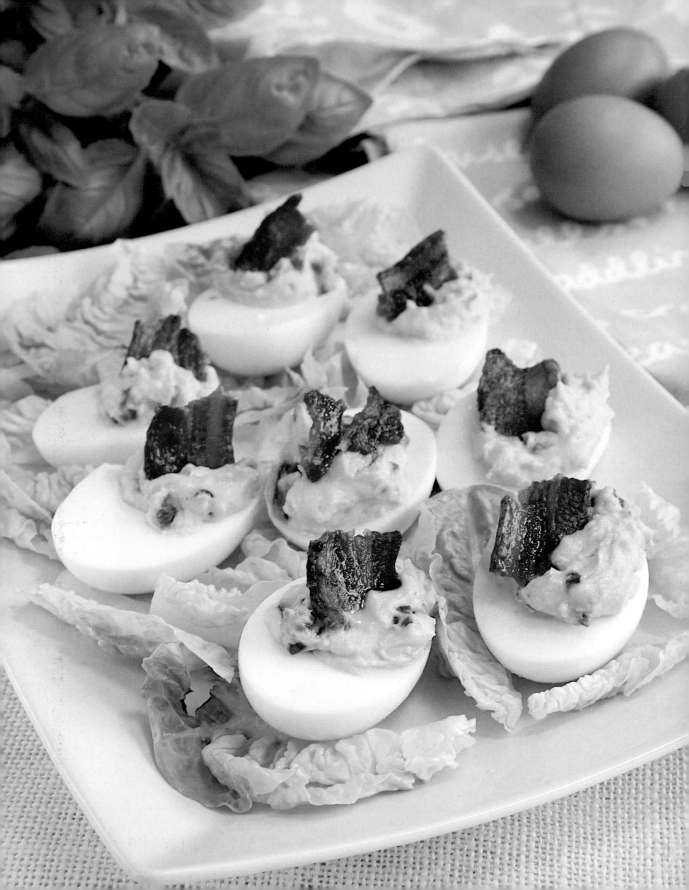

BACON DEVILED EGGS

Bacon and eggs aren't just for breakfast! These deviled eggs are a classic keto snack for any time of day.

4 SERVINGS	10 MINS	20 MINS

INGREDIENTS

Water

4 large pastured eggs

3 large slices (90 g/3.2 oz) of bacon

½ teaspoon salt

Freshly ground black pepper

¼ cup (55 g/1.9 oz) mayonnaise

NUTRITION FACTS PER SERVING
(2 deviled eggs)

Total carbs: 0.6 g

Fiber: 0.1 g

Net carbs: 0.6 g

Protein: 9.5 g

Fat: 21.8 g

Energy: 237 kcal

Macronutrient ratio:
Calories from carbs (1%), protein (16%), fat (83%)

Preheat the oven to 375°F (190°C, or gas mark 5). Fill a small saucepan up to three-quarters full with water. Hard boil the eggs and then transfer them to a bowl filled with cold water.

Meanwhile, lay the bacon on a cooking rack and set it on a tray to collect the bacon grease. Place the tray in the oven and cook for about 10 to 15 minutes until the bacon is browned. (The total cooking time depends on the thickness of the bacon slices.)

Halve the eggs lengthwise. Scoop the egg yolks into a small bowl and set the empty egg whites aside. Add the bacon grease to the yolks, season with salt and black pepper, and then mash the yolks with a fork. Add the mayonnaise. Crumble the bacon into the bowl and mix well. Keep some bacon aside for garnish. Top the egg white halves with the egg yolk mixture and the remaining bacon and serve the eggs by themselves or on top of lettuce leaves.

CURRIED COCONUT CHIPS

Trust me: you'll totally fall in love with these keto-friendly chips.
They make a super snack when you're trying to avoid sweet treats.

4 SERVINGS	5 MINS	10 MINS

INGREDIENTS

2 tablespoons (30 ml/1 fl oz) extra virgin coconut oil, melted

1 teaspoon curry powder

1 teaspoon garlic powder

¼ teaspoon cayenne pepper

½ teaspoon salt

2 cups (120 g/4.2 oz) desiccated coconut, flaked

NUTRITION FACTS PER SERVING

Total carbs: 8 g

Fiber: 5.2 g

Net carbs: 2.9 g

Protein: 2.3 g

Fat: 26.3 g

Energy: 261 kcal

Macronutrient ratio:
Calories from carbs (4%), protein (4%), fat (92%)

Preheat the oven to 350°F (175 °C, or gas mark 4). In a bowl, mix the melted coconut oil with the spices and salt and then stir in the flaked coconut. Spread the coated coconut on a baking sheet lined with parchment paper and bake for 4 to 7 minutes. (Keep an eye on the coconut: it burns easily, and if you cook it too long, it may become bitter.) When done, remove from the oven and set aside to cool. Store at room temperature in an airtight container for up to a month.

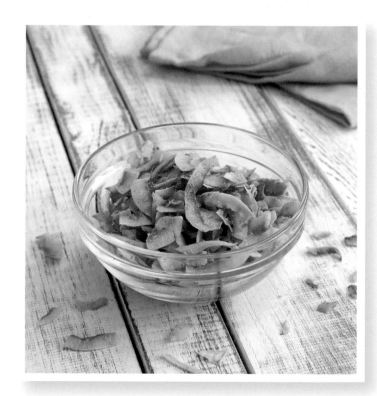

ONION & POPPY SEED CRACKERS

Dip these flavorful keto crackers into guacamole, sour cream, or pâté if you're after a quick bite on the run!

16 CRACKERS	15 MINS	20 MINS + CHILLING

INGREDIENTS

2 cups (200 g/7.1 oz) almond flour

⅓ cup (40 g/1.4 oz) coconut flour

2 tablespoons (18 g/0.6 oz) poppy seeds

1 teaspoon salt

1 medium (110 g/3.9 oz) onion

1 large pastured egg

Optional: ⅔ cup (60 g/2.1 oz) Parmesan cheese

NUTRITION FACTS PER CRACKER

Total carbs: 4 g

Fiber: 2 g

Net carbs: 2 g

Protein: 3.8 g

Fat: 7.7 g

Energy: 96 kcal

Macronutrient ratio: Calories from carbs (9%), protein (16%), fat (75%)

Mix all the dry ingredients in a bowl. Drop the onion into a blender and pulse until smooth. Add the onion, egg, and Parmesan cheese (if using) to the dry mixture and combine well. Flatten the dough in your hands and set in the fridge for 30 to 60 minutes.

Preheat the oven to 400°F (200°C, or gas mark 6). Remove the dough from the fridge and place it between two pieces of parchment paper or aluminum foil. Roll it out or press it down with your fingers into an 8 × 12 inch (20 × 30 cm) baking sheet.

Using a pizza cutter or sharp knife, cut the dough into 16 equal pieces and then place the sheet in the oven for 12 to 15 minutes. When done, remove from the oven and set aside to cool. Try the crackers with Smokey Fish Pâté (page 77) or Keto Hummus (page 71).

TIP

The crackers will be slightly chewy. If you prefer them crispier, use ¾ cup (75 g/2.7 oz) of almond flour or flax meal instead of the coconut flour. Alternatively, bake them for an additional 20 to 30 minutes on low (225°F/110°C).

PESTO CRACKERS

Use your favorite pesto sauce to make your own version of these savory, chewy crackers.

 16 CRACKERS   15 MINS   20 MINS + CHILLING

INGREDIENTS

2 cups (200 g/7.1 oz) almond flour

⅓ cup (40 g/1.4 oz) coconut flour

¼ cup (30 g/1.1 oz) chia seeds, ground

½ teaspoon salt

1 large pastured egg white

½ cup (125 g/4.4 oz) red or other pesto sauce

Optional: ⅔ cup (60 g/2.1 oz) Parmesan cheese

NUTRITION FACTS PER CRACKER

Total carbs: 4.4 g

Fiber: 2.6 g

Net carbs: 1.8 g

Protein: 4 g

Fat: 11.5 g

Energy: 130 kcal

Macronutrient ratio:
Calories from carbs (5%), protein (13%), fat (82%)

Mix all the dry ingredients in a bowl. Add the egg white, pesto sauce, and Parmesan cheese (if using) to the dry mixture and combine well. Flatten the dough in your hands and place in the fridge for 30 to 60 minutes.

Preheat the oven to 400°F (200°C, or gas mark 6). Remove the dough from the fridge and set it between two pieces of parchment paper or aluminum foil. Roll it out or press it down with your fingers into an 8 × 12 inch (20 × 30 cm) baking sheet.

Using a pizza cutter or sharp knife, cut the dough into 16 equal pieces and bake for 12 to 15 minutes. When done, remove from the oven and set aside to cool. Enjoy the crackers with Smokey Fish Pâté (opposite) or Keto Hummus (page 71).

TIP

These crackers will be slightly chewy. If you prefer them crispier, use ¾ cup (75 g/2.7 oz) of almond flour or flax meal instead of the coconut flour. Alternatively, bake for an additional 20 to 30 minutes on low (225°F/110°C).

SMOKY FISH PÂTÉ

This easy-to-make fish pâté is just loaded with healthy omega-3 fatty acids.

 8 SERVINGS | **5 MINS** | **5 MINS**

INGREDIENTS

1 medium (100 g/3.5 oz) red onion

1 package (100 g/3.5 oz) smoked salmon

1 large (200 g/7.1 oz) smoked mackerel filet

3.5 ounces (100 g) cream cheese

½ cup (115 g/4.1 oz) sour cream

2 tablespoons (30 ml/1 fl oz) fresh lemon juice

Freshly ground black pepper, to taste

NUTRITION FACTS PER SERVING

Total carbs: 2 g

Fiber: 0.2 g

Net carbs: 1.8 g

Protein: 8.3 g

Fat: 10.4 g

Energy: 129 kcal

Macronutrient ratio: Calories from carbs (5%), protein (25%), fat (70%)

Peel and finely chop the onion. Put the smoked salmon and mackerel into a blender together with the cream cheese and sour cream and then pulse until smooth. Add the lemon juice and season with black pepper. Add the onion and pulse just enough to mix it in. (Don't blend it in completely: leave some small pieces in the mixture.) Serve with freshly-cut vegetables or as a topping for Ultimate Keto Bread (page 19), Onion & Poppy Seed Crackers (page 75), or Pesto Crackers (page 77).

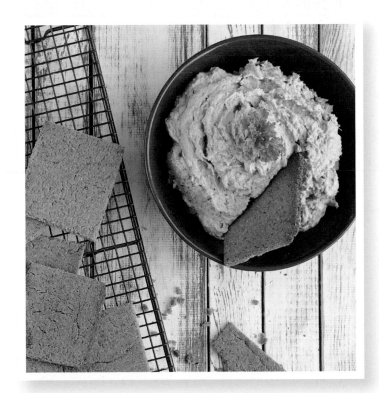

Chapter Five:

HEALTHY LUNCH IDEAS

It's 1 p.m., and breakfast seems like an awfully long time ago. Your stomach is rumbling, and that means you need a satiating meal that has the staying power to see you through till dinner. What do you do? Try some of the low-carb recipes in this chapter! From grain-free sandwiches to salmon nori rolls and keto-friendly protein bars, here are some of my favorite ways to enjoy a healthy lunch. And lots of these recipes can do double duty, too: they also make great light dinners.

VEGETABLE FRITTERS

I can't get enough of these vegetable fritters. They make a nice light lunch or side dish: serve them with guacamole, sour cream, or my Spicy Chocolate BBQ Sauce for dipping.

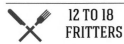 12 TO 18 FRITTERS	15 MINS	45 TO 50 MINS

INGREDIENTS

1 small (60 g/2.1 oz) red onion

1 large (200 g/7.1 oz) turnip

1 small (200 g/7.1 oz) celeriac

2 medium (400 g/14.1 oz) zucchini

½ teaspoon salt

¼ cup (55 g/1.9 oz) ghee or coconut oil, melted

⅓ cup (50 g/1.8 oz) flax meal

1 teaspoon garlic powder

1 teaspoon turmeric

2 large pastured eggs

Optional: ¼ cup (25 g/0.9 oz) Parmesan or shredded cheddar cheese or 4 slices crispy bacon

NUTRITION FACTS PER SERVING

(2 to 3 fritters)

Total carbs: 11.2 g

Fiber: 4.4 g

Net carbs: 6.8 g

Protein: 5.5 g

Fat: 14.7 g

Energy: 193 kcal

Macronutrient ratio:
Calories from carbs (15%), protein (12%), fat (73%)

Preheat the oven to 400°F (200°C, or gas mark 6). Line a baking sheet with parchment paper. (Alternatively, you can fry the fritters in a pan greased with ghee.)

Peel the onion, turnips, and celeriac. Wash and leave the skin on the zucchini. Slice the onion. Using a julienne peeler, vegetable spiralizer, or a regular grater, shred the celeriac, turnips, and zucchini into thin "noodles."

Combine all the vegetables into a mixing bowl and season with salt. Set aside for 20 minutes to let the vegetables release their juices. Then pat dry with a paper towel.

Add the melted ghee or coconut oil (if frying, pour into the pan instead), as well as the flax meal, garlic powder, turmeric, eggs, and Parmesan cheese or bacon (if using). Season with salt again and mix well. Begin assembling medium-sized fritters on the baking sheet; you should have about 12 to 18 fritters. Place the fritters in the oven and bake for about 15 to 20 minutes.

When done, the fritters should be crispy and lightly browned on top. Remove from the oven and set aside to cool.

SALMON & SPINACH ROULADE

Salmon and spinach work so well together, especially in this light lunch that's packed with healthy omega-3 fatty acids. It makes an impressive party snack, too!

4 SERVINGS	15 MINS	30 MINS

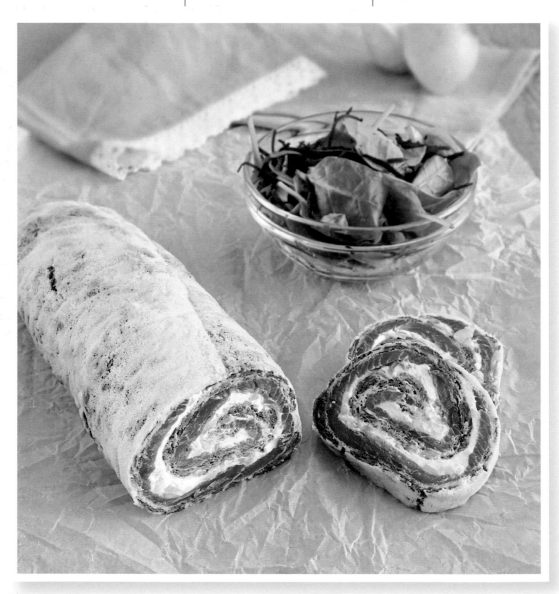

INGREDIENTS

2 tablespoons (30 g/1.1 oz) ghee or butter

1 clove garlic, crushed

1 large package spinach, fresh (250 g/8.8 oz) or frozen (275 g/ 9.7 oz)

4 large eggs

¼ teaspoon salt

¼ teaspoon cream of tartar

5.3 ounces (150 g) cream cheese

¼ cup (60 g/2.1 oz) sour cream

1 tablespoon (15 ml/0.5 fl oz) fresh lemon juice

2 medium (30 g/1.1 oz) spring onions or chives,

2 packages (200 g/7.1 oz) smoked salmon

NUTRITION FACTS PER SERVING

Total carbs: 5.4 g

Fiber: 1.7 g

Net carbs: 3.7 g

Protein: 20.3 g

Fat: 28.1 g

Energy: 337 kcal

Macronutrient ratio: Calories from carbs (4%), protein (23%), fat (73%)

Preheat the oven to 375°F (190°C, or gas mark 5). Line a baking sheet or a Swiss roll pan with parchment paper. Wash and dry the spinach if using fresh. In a large pan, heat the ghee over medium heat and add the crushed garlic. Cook for one minute and then add the spinach. Cook for another minute until wilted (or, if using frozen spinach, until it's defrosted.) Remove from the heat and set aside. Once cooled, pour off any excess juices.

To make the roulade, separate the egg whites from the egg yolks. In one bowl, beat the egg yolks. In a separate bowl, beat the egg whites with the salt and cream of tartar until they create soft peaks. Next, slowly mix in the whisked egg yolks. Be gentle: don't deflate the egg whites while folding in the egg yolks.

Slowly fold the eggs into the spinach mixture: start by combining just a few tablespoons (45 to 55 g/1.6 to 1.9 oz) with the spinach and then mix in the remaining eggs.

Place the mixture in the parchment paper-lined tray and spread evenly. Bake for 10 to 12 minutes until it firms up and the top is lightly browned. Remove from the oven and cover with a damp kitchen towel until cool. This will prevent the eggs from getting too dry and will make the rolling easier.

Meanwhile, prepare the filling. Mix the cream cheese, sour cream, lemon juice, and finely chopped spring onion or chives. Season with a pinch of salt and mix well.

Flip the roulade onto a cutting board. Peel off the parchment paper and start adding the filling: Lay the pieces of smoked salmon all over the roulade, leaving small gaps on all sides. Spread the cream cheese filling over the salmon and then roll up the roulade tightly. Serve immediately by cutting into slices or wrap in aluminum foil and keep refrigerated.

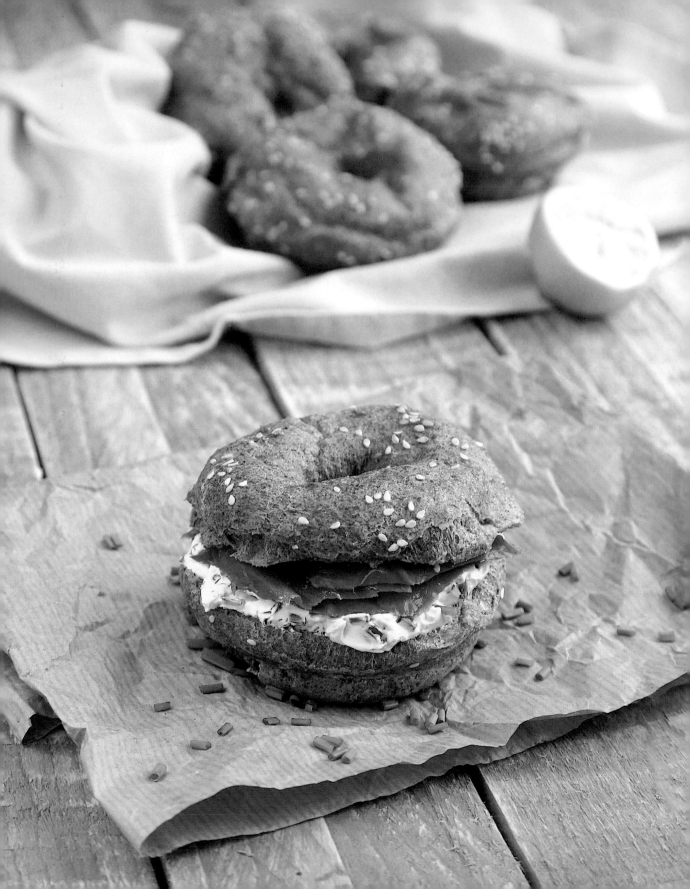

HEALTHY SALMON BAGELS

This convenient, keto-friendly lunch can be made in advance, then snatched from the fridge as you're running out the door in the morning.

 2 SERVINGS | **5 MINS** | **5 MINS**

INGREDIENTS

2 Ultimate Keto Buns (page 26)

2.1 ounces (60 g) cream cheese

2 tablespoons (30 g/1.1 oz) mayonnaise

2 tablespoons (6 g/0.2 oz) chopped chives

1 tablespoon (4 g/0.14 oz) chopped fresh dill

1 tablespoon (15 ml/0.5 fl oz) fresh lemon juice

1 package (100 g/3.5 oz) smoked salmon

NUTRITION FACTS PER SERVING

Total carbs: 14.4 g

Fiber: 8.3 g

Net carbs: 6 g

Protein: 23.8 g

Fat: 54.2 g

Energy: 597 kcal

Macronutrient ratio: Calories from carbs (4%), protein (16%), fat (80%)

Follow the recipe for Ultimate Keto Buns, but shape the pieces into bagels or use a donut baking pan.

Mix together the cream cheese, mayonnaise, chives, and dill. Halve each bagel widthwise and spread the cream cheese mixture on each side. Drizzle the lemon juice over the smoked salmon and then place the fish on top of the cream cheese on two of the bagel halves. Close each sandwich and serve.

MEATY GUACMUFFINS

Muffins with meat? Yes, you heard that right! These hearty, savory muffins are even better when topped with a creamy guacamole "frosting."

12 MUFFINS	15 MINS	35 TO 40 MINS

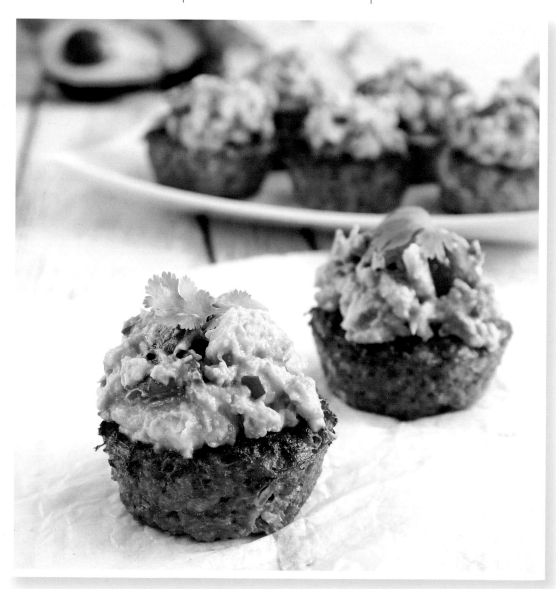

INGREDIENTS

2 tablespoons (30 g/1.1oz) ghee or lard

2 cloves garlic, crushed

1 small (70 g/2.5 oz) white onion, diced

2½ cups (300 g/10.6 oz) Cauli-Rice (page 37)

1.1 pound (500 g/17.6 oz) beef, ground

2 large eggs

2 teaspoons paprika

1 teaspoon Dijon Mustard (page 31)

½ teaspoon salt

Guacamole "Frosting"
1½ medium (300 g/10.6 oz) avocados

1 small (70 g/2.5 oz) white onion, finely chopped

2 tablespoons (30 ml/1 fl oz) freshly squeezed lime juice

1 cup (150 g/5.3 oz) cherry tomatoes, coarsely chopped

2 tablespoons (2 g/0.07 oz) chopped cilantro

1 small hot chile pepper, chopped

2 cloves garlic

Salt and freshly ground black pepper, to taste

Preheat the oven to 350°F (175°C, or gas mark 4).

Heat the ghee in a large pan and add the crushed garlic and finely diced onion. Cook for 3 to 5 minutes and then add the Cauli-Rice. Cook for about 10 minutes, stirring frequently. Season with salt and set aside.

In a bowl, mix the ground beef, eggs, paprika, mustard, and Cauli-Rice mixture. Season with salt to taste and mix until well combined. Divide the meat mixture evenly between the cups of a muffin pan, place in the oven, and bake for 20 to 25 minutes until lightly browned and crispy on top. Remove from the oven and let cool.

Meanwhile, prepare the guacamole "frosting." Halve and peel the avocados, remove the stones, and put half of the avocado into a bowl. Mash it well with a fork. Add the finely chopped onion, lime juice, coarsely-chopped tomatoes, cilantro, chile pepper, and crushed garlic.

Dice the rest of the avocado and mix it into the salad, but do not mash it. Season with salt and black pepper to taste. Top each of the meat muffins with the guacamole and serve.

TIP

Using lime juice in your guac and keeping it in an airtight container will keep it a vibrant green for longer.

NUTRITION FACTS PER MUFFIN

Total carbs: 5.7 g	**Protein:** 9.6 g	**Macronutrient ratio:**
Fiber: 2.8 g	**Fat:** 15.5 g	Calories from carbs (6%), protein (20%), fat (74%)
Net carbs: 3 g	**Energy:** 197 kcal	

CHICKEN CHARD WRAPS

A lunchbox staple, these Chicken Chard Wraps are
sure to stave off hunger until dinnertime.

2 WRAPS	5 MINS	15 MINS

INGREDIENTS

Water

2 large eggs

2 medium (30 g/1.1 oz) spring
onions or chives

1 tablespoon (15 g/0.5 oz)
Dijon Mustard (page 31)

2 tablespoons (30 ml/1 fl oz)
freshly squeezed lemon juice

3 tablespoons (45 g/1.6 oz)
Mayonnaise (page 28)

Salt and freshly ground black
pepper, to taste

2 cups (250 g/8.8 oz) Simple
Shredded Chicken (page 128)

4 to 8 large (180 g/6.3 oz)
chard leaves

NUTRITION FACTS
PER SERVING

Total carbs: 6.4 g

Fiber: 2.1 g

Net carbs: 4.3 g

Protein: 32.1 g

Fat: 44 g

Energy: 545 kcal

Macronutrient ratio:
Calories from carbs (3%),
protein (24%), fat (73%)

First, hardboil the eggs. Next, chop the spring onions and place
in a bowl of water: any dirt on the onion will settle at the bottom
of the bowl. Remove the onions and drain well on a paper towel.
Mix the spring onion with the mustard, lemon juice, and mayo.
Season with salt and black pepper. Wash the chard leaves.

Place the Simple Shredded Chicken on top of the chard leaves.
Top with the mayo dressing and sliced hard-boiled egg. Wrap the
chard around the filling and eat immediately.

TIP

You can prepare healthy chard wraps in the evening and have them
ready to take to work in refrigerated lunch boxes. Simply fill the chard
with some protein (eggs, chicken, tuna, salmon, etc.) and add homemade
mayo, cream cheese, shredded cheese, and your favorite spices and
herbs—the options are endless!

EASY CLOUD SANDWICHES

As light and fluffy as their name suggests, these grain-free sandwiches are ideal for a quick, keto-friendly lunch.

2 SANDWICHES	10 MINS	15 MINS

INGREDIENTS

Sandwich Buns

2 large eggs, separated

Pinch of salt

¼ teaspoon cream of tartar

⅔ cup (60 g/2.1 oz) grated Parmesan or cheddar cheese

Filling

2 tablespoons (30 g/1.1 oz) butter

¼ cup (50 g/1.8 oz) cream cheese

4 slices (100 g/3.5 oz) high-quality ham

2 slices (56 g/2 oz) cheddar or Swiss cheese

4 leaves (40 g/1.4 oz) lettuce

NUTRITION FACTS PER SERVING

Total carbs: 3.5 g

Fiber: 0.3 g

Net carbs: 3.2 g

Protein: 34.3 g

Fat: 42.1 g

Energy: 520 kcal

Macronutrient ratio: Calories from carbs (2%), protein (26%), fat (72%)

Preheat the oven to 450°F (230°C, or gas mark 8). Separate the egg whites from the egg yolks and reserve the yolks. Add the salt and cream of tartar to the egg whites and whip them into a thick foam using a whisk or a food processor.

Gently fold the Parmesan cheese into the whisked egg whites with a spoon. (For a dairy-free bun, use finely chopped crispy bacon, ham, or fresh herbs like parsley, basil, or chives in place of the Parmesan cheese.) Whisk the egg yolks and slowly mix them into the egg whites. Be gentle: don't deflate the egg whites.

Line a baking sheet with parchment paper. Using a spoon, create four mounds of the fluffy egg mixture. Bake in the oven for about 3 minutes. Lower the temperature to 400°F (200°C, or gas mark 6) and bake for another 10 minutes. Remove from the oven and set aside to cool. Top with butter, cream cheese, ham, cheddar cheese, and lettuce or try some of the following options.

TIPS FOR OTHER FILLINGS (PER SERVING)

Tuna melt: 2 ounces (56 g) canned tuna, 2 tablespoons (30 g/1.1 oz) mayo, 1 small spring onion, 1 tablespoon (15 ml/0.5 fl oz) lemon juice, ¼ cup (30 g/1.1 oz) shredded cheddar cheese

Tandoori chicken: 3 ounces (85 g) shredded chicken, 2 lettuce leaves, 2 tablespoons (30 g/1.1 oz) full-fat yogurt, and 1 teaspoon tandoori spice mix

Pork & slaw: 3 ounces (85 g) Perfectly Pulled Pork (page 163), ½ serving Creamy Keto Coleslaw (page 105)

SALMON NORI ROLLS

These Salmon Nori Rolls make excellent workday lunches or party snacks. You'll definitely want to make enough to share!

 4 SERVINGS | **15 MINS** | **20 MINS**

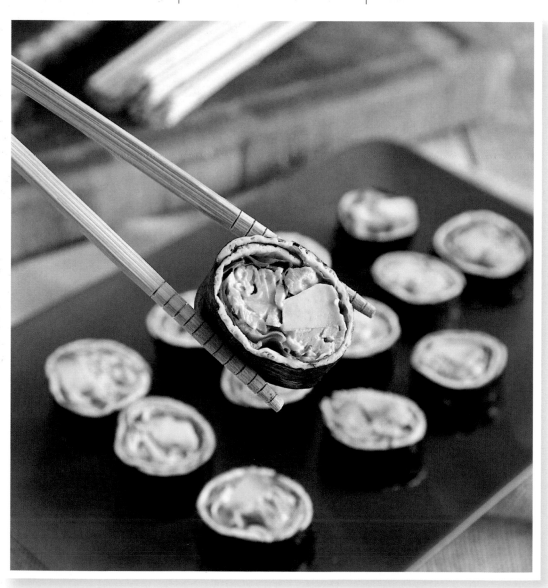

INGREDIENTS

Nori rolls

2 medium (300 g/10.6 oz) salmon fillets

½ teaspoon salt, divided

2 tablespoons (30 ml/1 fl oz) freshly squeezed lemon juice

1 tablespoon (15 g/0.5 oz) ghee or coconut oil

4 large eggs

¼ cup (55 g/1.9 oz) Spicy Mayonnaise (recipe below)

4 nori seaweed sheets

4 cups (120 g/4.2 oz) lettuce leaves

1 large (200 g/7.1 oz) avocado

2 tablespoons (8 g/0.3 oz) chopped fresh dill

Spicy Mayonnaise

½ cup (110 g/3.9 oz) Mayonnaise (page 28)

2 tablespoons (30 ml/1.1 fl oz) Sriracha or hot sauce

NUTRITION FACTS PER SERVING

(1 uncut roll)

Total carbs: 8.5 g

Fiber: 4.7 g

Net carbs: 3.8 g

Protein: 25.3 g

Fat: 43.4 g

Energy: 516 kcal

Macronutrient ratio: Calories from carbs (3%), protein (20%), fat (77%)

First, cook the salmon. Fill a steaming pot with about 2 inches (5 cm) of water. Bring to a boil over high heat.

Season the salmon fillets with a pinch of the salt and drizzle with half the lemon juice. Reduce the heat to medium and place in the salmon in a steaming basket. Cover with a lid and cook for 8 to 10 minutes or until the fish is opaque and separates easily when pierced with a fork.

Meanwhile, prepare the egg omelets. Grease a pan with some of the ghee. Crack an egg into a small bowl and season with a pinch of the salt. Mix well with a fork and pour the mixture into the hot pan. Spread the egg as evenly as possible over the surface of the pan to make a thin omelet: it doesn't need to be round in shape. Cook until the top is firm. Remove from the pan and set on a plate. Repeat with the remaining eggs; grease the pan again if needed.

Prepare the Spicy Mayonnaise by mixing the mayonnaise with the Sriracha.

When the salmon is cooked, remove the skin and crumble the flesh into a bowl. Add half of the Spicy Mayonnaise and the chopped dill and mix until well combined. Keep the remaining Spicy Mayonnaise for later.

Start assembling the roll. Place an egg omelet on top of a nori sheet. Make sure the omelet doesn't cover the whole nori sheet; leave 1 to 2 inches (2.5 to 5 cm) on the sides so you can seal the nori roll. If the omelet is too big, cut the edges and put the cuttings in the middle of the roll.

Top each with 1 cup (30 g/1.1 oz) of lettuce, ¼ of the sliced avocado, and ¼ of the salmon mixture. Make sure you place the filling only on the first half of the omelet so you can wrap it easily. Roll it up, wet the free nori edge with a few drops of water, and seal well. Set the roll on a plate with the sealed side down to keep it tight. Repeat with the remaining ingredients. Leave to rest for 10 to 15 minutes before serving or put it in the fridge. Cut each roll into 8 pieces and serve with the remaining Spicy Mayonnaise.

REUBEN SANDWICH

Who could say no to this keto-friendly version of the classic Reuben sandwich? It's an irresistible combination of sauerkraut, pastrami, Swiss cheese, and Russian dressing.

2 SANDWICHES	10 MINS	15 MINS

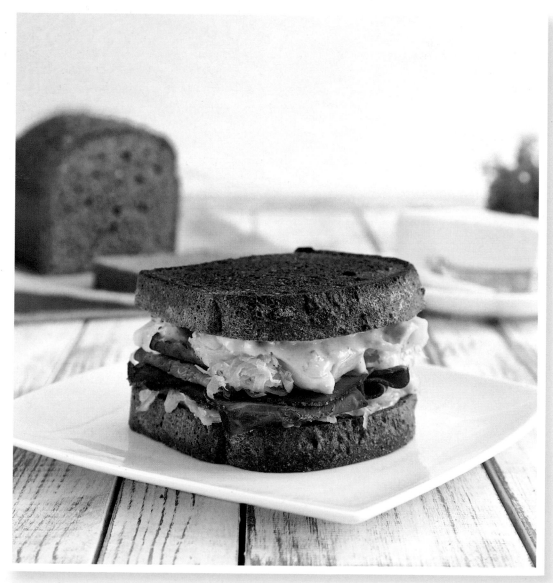

INGREDIENTS

Russian Dressing

1 small (40 g/1.4 oz) pickle

½ teaspoon grated horseradish

3 tablespoons (45 g/1.6 oz) Mayonnaise (page 28)

1 tablespoon (15 g/0.5 oz) sour cream or more mayonnaise

1 teaspoon Sriracha or hot sauce

1 medium (15 g/0.5 oz) spring onion or chives

1 tablespoon (15 ml/0.5 fl oz) freshly squeezed lemon juice

1 tablespoon (4 g/0.14 oz) chopped fresh parsley

Salt to taste

Sandwich

2 tablespoons (30 g/1.1 oz) butter or ghee

4 slices Ultimate Keto Bread (page 19)

2 slices (56 g/2 oz) Swiss cheese

½ cup (75 g/2.6 oz) sauerkraut

4 slices (80 g/2.8 oz) pastrami or corned beef

NUTRITION FACTS PER SANDWICH

Total carbs: 21.8 g

Fiber: 14.6 g

Net carbs: 7.2 g

Protein: 34.9 g

Fat: 64.5 g

Energy: 752 kcal

Macronutrient ratio: Calories from carbs (4%), protein (19%), fat (77%)

First, make the Russian dressing. Grate the pickle and peel and grate the horseradish. Put them in a bowl with the remaining ingredients for the dressing, mix, and set aside.

Spread ½ tablespoon (7.5 g/0.3 oz) of butter or ghee on each bread slice. Turn the slices over and spread half of the Russian dressing on the other side.

Over two slices, spread half of the cheese, half of the sauerkraut, and all of the pastrami. Spread the remaining Russian dressing over the pastrami and top with the remaining sauerkraut and cheese. Place the remaining slice of bread on top, with the buttered side up.

Heat a regular or a griddle pan over a medium-high heat. Place the sandwich in the pan and press down on it with a spatula. (Alternatively, you can use a sandwich press.) Cook for about 5 minutes on each side until the bread is crispy and browned and the cheese starts to melt. When done, serve immediately.

TIP

For a lighter option, substitute the Ultimate Keto Bread with Fluffy Grain-Free Sunflower Bread (page 28).

ZUCCHINI LASAGNA

This lighter version of everyone's favorite Italian dish will help you stay fuller for longer. It has a bit of a Greek twist, too, since it uses lamb instead of beef.

4 SERVINGS	10 MINS	35 TO 40 MINS

INGREDIENTS

2 tablespoons (30 g/1.1 oz) ghee

2 cloves garlic, crushed

1.3 pounds (600 g) lamb, ground

2 teaspoons oregano, dried

2 teaspoons basil, dried

1 tablespoon (7 g/0.25 oz) paprika

½ teaspoon salt

4 medium (800 g/1.7 lb) zucchini

1 cup (240 g/8.5 oz) canned diced tomatoes

⅔ cup (60 g/2.1 oz) Parmesan cheese, grated

NUTRITION FACTS PER SERVING

Total carbs: 11.3 g

Fiber: 3.8 g

Net carbs: 7.5 g

Protein: 34.5 g

Fat: 43.4 g

Energy: 563 kcal

Macronutrient ratio:
Calories from carbs (5%), protein (25%), fat (70%)

Heat a large pan greased with ghee and add the crushed garlic. Cook for one minute and then add the ground lamb, dried oregano, basil, paprika, and salt. Mix and cook until the meat is browned on all sides. When done, remove from the heat and set aside.

Preheat the oven to 400°F (200°C, or gas mark 6). Meanwhile, prepare the zucchini. Wash the zucchini and use a potato peeler or a sharp knife to thinly slice the zucchini into wide "noodles." Lay a third of the zucchini slices in a large caserole dish and top with half of the meat mixture. Add a third of the Parmesan cheese, then another layer of zucchini slices. Add the remaining layer of the meat mixture and top with more Parmesan and the last layer of the zucchini slices.

Sprinkle the top of the lasagna with the remaining Parmesan cheese and place in the oven. Cook for 25 to 30 minutes. When done, remove from the oven and set aside to cool for 10 minutes. Enjoy immediately or refrigerate when completely cool and store for up to 3 days.

BACON-WRAPPED LIVER PÂTÉ

Even if you think you don't like offal, you're still going to love this recipe. Chicken liver has a milder taste and goes surprisingly well with crispy bacon. I like adding these to green salads or serving them as hors d'oeuvres at parties.

 4 SERVINGS | **15 MINS** | **40 TO 45 MINS**

INGREDIENTS

1 pound (450 g) chicken liver

¼ cup ghee or lard (56 g/2 oz)

1 medium white onion (110 g/3.9 oz), peeled and finely chopped

2 cloves garlic, peeled and crushed

½ small celeriac (100 g/3.5 oz), peeled

8 slices (120 g/4.2 oz) of thinly-cut bacon

Salt and freshly ground black pepper, to taste

NUTRITION FACTS PER SERVING

Total carbs: 6.2 g

Fiber: 1 g

Net carbs: 5.2 g

Protein: 23.9 g

Fat: 26.8 g

Energy: 366 kcal

Macronutrient ratio:
Calories from carbs (6%), protein (27%), fat (67%)

Preheat the oven to 325°F (160°C, or gas mark 3). Chop the chicken livers into small pieces. Heat half of the ghee in a pan and add the livers. Cook for just about 3 minutes until the livers are browned on the outsides but still pink inside. Transfer the livers to a blender and pulse until smooth.

Place the remaining ghee into a clean pan and add the onion, garlic, and celeriac. Cook over a medium heat for about 10 minutes, stirring frequently.

Add the cooked onion-celeriac mixture to the pureed chicken livers in the blender and pulse until smooth. For a chunkier texture, reserve some of the cooked vegetables to add in after blending.

Cut the bacon slices lengthwise into 16 slices. Season the liver mixture with salt and black pepper to taste and use a spoon to form it into small ovals. Place an oval on a slice of bacon and wrap the bacon around the pâté to create 16 small parcels. Transfer to a baking sheet and cook for 25 to 30 minutes.

When done, remove from the oven and set aside. Serve warm or at room temperature, in salads or on their own.

SPICED COCONUT GRANOLA BARS

These granola bars are so filling: they're standalone meals in themselves.
Keep a few in the car or in your bag in case you need an on-the-go snack.

8 SERVINGS	10 MINS	30 MINS

INGREDIENTS

½ cup (35 g/1.2 oz) each unsweetened dried shredded coconut and flaked coconut

¼ cup (35 g/1.2 oz) each almonds, macadamia nuts, pecans, chia seeds and pumpkin seeds

⅓ cup (35 g/1.2 oz) whey protein or egg white protein powder

1 tablespoon (7 g/0.25 oz) pumpkin-spice mix

¼ cup (40 g/1.4 oz) erythritol, powdered

Pinch salt

2 large egg whites

¾ cup (185 g/6.6 oz) coconut butter or Toasted Nut Butter (page 39)

2 tablespoons (30 g/1.1 oz) extra virgin coconut oil or butter

½ cup (120 ml/4.2 fl oz) coconut milk

15 to 20 drops liquid stevia

Preheat the oven to 325°F (160°C, or gas mark 3). Place the shredded and flaked coconut in a large mixing bowl. Roughly chop the almonds, macadamia nuts, and pecans. Add the nuts, then the chia and pumpkin seeds, protein powder (plain or vanilla), pumpkin spice mix, powdered erythritol, and salt. Mix until well combined.

Put the egg whites, coconut butter (or Toasted Nut Butter), coconut oil, coconut milk, and liquid stevia into a small saucepan and gently heat until melted and combined. Pour the coconut mixture into the dry mixture and combine well.

Line an 8 × 8 inch (20 × 20 cm) pan with parchment paper or use a silicone pan. Scoop the mixture into the dish and spread it out evenly using a spatula. Bake for about 30 minutes. When done, remove the dish from the oven and place it on a rack to cool. Let the granola cool completely before cutting into 8 bars. Store at room temperature in an airtight container for up to 5 days or refrigerate for up to 10 days.

TIP

You can make your own pumpkin spice mix. To get ½ cup (48 g/1.7 oz) pumpkin pie spice mix, combine ¼ cup (28 g/1 oz) Ceylon cinnamon, 2 tablespoons (11 g/0.4 oz) ground ginger, 2 teaspoons ground nutmeg, 1 teaspoon ground cloves, and 1 teaspoon ground allspice. Optionally, add ½ teaspoon ground cardamom and ½ teaspoon ground mace. Store in an airtight container in your cupboard.

NUTRITION FACTS PER SERVING

Total carbs: 12.7 g	**Protein:** 11.3 g	**Macronutrient ratio:** Calories from carbs (5%), protein (12%), fat (83%)
Fiber: 8.5 g	**Fat:** 33.9 g	
Net carbs: 4.2 g	**Energy:** 377 kcal	

FUDGY PROTEIN BARS

These chocolatey keto bars are some of the best I've ever created.
They're super-easy to prepare, and they're so filling!

 8 SERVINGS | **10 MINS** | **10 MINS** + CHILLING

INGREDIENTS

1 recipe (about 500 g/17.6 oz) Chocolate Hazelnut Butter (page 43), at room temperature

1 cup (100 g/3.5 oz) whey protein or egg white protein powder

½ cup (50 g/1.8 oz) almond flour

Optional: 10 to 15 drops liquid stevia

2 tablespoons (28 g/1 oz) cacao nibs or dark chocolate, 85% cacao or more, chopped

NUTRITION FACTS PER SERVING

Total carbs: 14.4 g

Fiber: 7 g

Net carbs: 7.4 g

Protein: 19.3 g

Fat: 41.4 g

Energy: 476 kcal

Macronutrient ratio: Calories from carbs (6%), protein (16%), fat (78%)

Place the Chocolate Hazelnut Butter in a bowl. Add the whey protein, almond flour, and liquid stevia (if using). Mix until everything is well combined.

Line an 8 × 8 inch (20 × 20 cm) pan with parchment paper or use a silicone pan. Scoop the mixture into the dish and spread it evenly using a spatula. Sprinkle with cacao nibs or chopped dark chocolate. Place in the fridge for up to 2 hours or until set. Use a pizza cutter to slice into 8 bars. Keep refrigerated so the bars won't melt. Store in the fridge for up to 10 days.

TIP

Coconut oil and nut butters soften at room temperature, so make sure you keep your keto meals refrigerated. If you take the bars to work, make sure you place them in a secure container and get them back in the fridge as soon as possible.

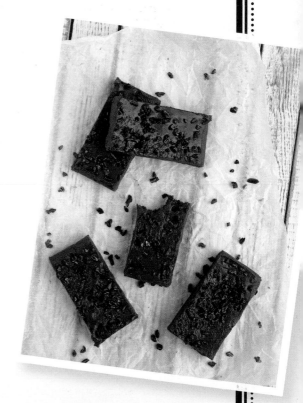

Chapter Six:

SATISFYING SOUPS & SALADS

When you're following a low-carb diet, it's so important to eat plenty of nutrient-dense food, such as vegetables, avocados, meat, and nuts. That'll help you stave off hunger pangs and overcome sugar cravings—and so will the recipes in this chapter. From crunchy Caesar salad served in homemade cheese "bowls" to creamy green gazpacho and a stick-to-your-ribs chicken minestrone, these soups and salads are great on their own as healthy, work-friendly lunches or as light dinners, but they also work well as starters or side dishes for larger, longer meals.

CREAMY GREEN GAZPACHO

This cold, refreshing soup is high in potassium, and it's just
what you want for a light lunch on a hot summer's day.

4 SERVINGS	10 MINS	10 MINS

INGREDIENTS

2 large (400 g/14.1 oz) avocados

1 large (300 g/10.6 oz)
cucumber

1 large (160 g/5.6 oz)
green pepper

1 medium (110 g/3.9 oz)
white onion

2 cloves garlic, crushed

1 (15 g/0.5 oz) jalapeño
pepper, deseeded

Juice from 1 lime

2 to 4 tablespoons (2 to 4 g/
0.07 to 0.1 oz) chopped
cilantro, to taste

½ cup (120 ml/4 fl oz)
extra virgin olive oil

Salt and freshly ground black
pepper, to taste

Optional: 1 cup (230 g/8.2 oz)
sour cream or full-fat yogurt

Halve the avocado and remove the pit. Peel and slice it and
place it in a blender. Wash, peel, and slice the cucumber. Wash,
halve, and deseed the green bell pepper and then slice it into
strips. Add both to the blender with the avocado.

Peel and roughly chop the onion and garlic, wash, halve and
deseed the jalapeño, and put everything into the blender. Add the
lime juice, cilantro, and olive oil. Save a little of the olive oil and
cilantro for garnish. Season with salt and black pepper.

Pulse all the ingredients until smooth. (You can use a hand
blender, too, but it will take longer to process.) Transfer to
a serving bowl and drizzle some olive oil on top. Add a dollop
of sour cream or full-fat yogurt for a touch of creaminess.

NUTRITION FACTS PER SERVING

Total carbs: 16.4 g	**Protein:** 3.3 g	**Macronutrient ratio:** Calories from carbs (7%), protein (3%), fat (90%)
Fiber: 8.6 g	**Fat:** 42.3 g	
Net carbs: 7.8 g	**Energy:** 438 kcal	

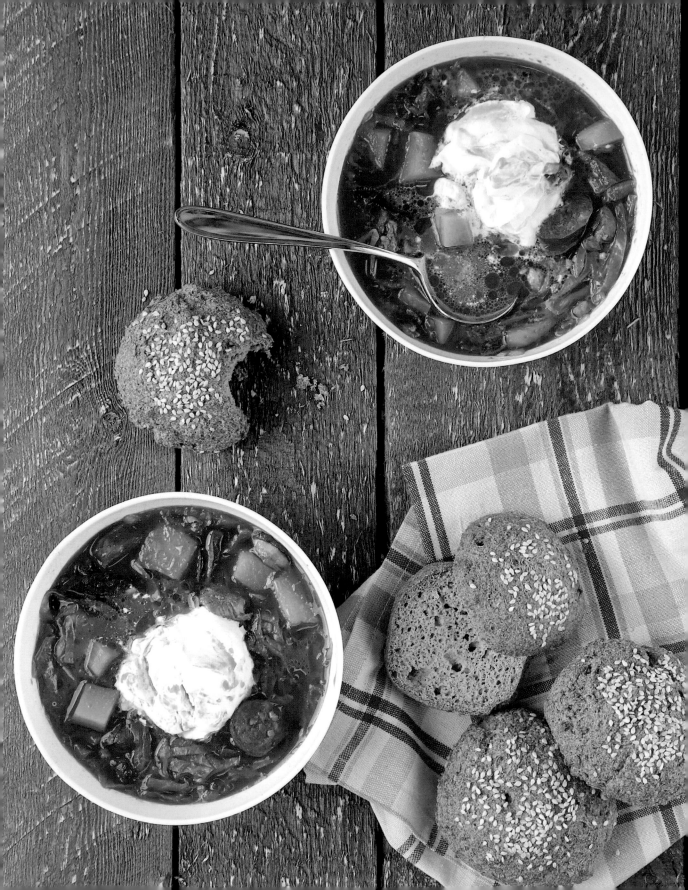

SLOVAK SAUERKRAUT SOUP

Based on a delicious soup made in Slovakia and the Czech Republic during the holiday season, this recipe is one of my absolute favorites! It's low-carb comfort food at its best.

 10 SERVINGS | **20 MINS** | **2 HOURS**

INGREDIENTS

1.3 pounds (600 g) pork shoulder

¼ cup (56 g/2 oz) ghee or lard

¼ teaspoon each ground cloves and nutmeg

1.3 pounds (600 g) sauerkraut

1½ cups (45 g/1.6 oz) wild mushrooms, dried

2 cloves garlic, crushed

2 tablespoons (30 g/1.1 oz) tomato puree, unsweetened

1 teaspoon each whole peppercorns and salt

1 tablespoon (7 g/0.24 oz) caraway seeds

4 bay leaves

2 cups (480 ml/16 fl oz) Bone Broth (page 30)

1½ quarts (1.5 L/50.7 fl oz) water

1 large (200 g/7.1 oz) Hungarian salami, sliced

1 medium (500 g/17.6 oz) rutabaga

Dice the pork into medium-sized pieces. Heat the ghee in a large pot and then add the pork, ground cloves, and nutmeg. Brown the meat on all sides, stirring frequently.

Add the sauerkraut, dried mushrooms, crushed garlic, tomato puree, peppercorns, caraway seeds, bay leaves, salt, Bone Broth, and water. Cover with a lid and let the mixture simmer for 60 to 75 minutes or until the sauerkraut is tender.

Slice the sausage. Peel and dice the rutabaga into medium pieces and set aside. Once the sauerkraut is tender, add the sausage and rutabaga and cook for another 15 to 20 minutes or until the rutabaga is tender. If using heavy whipping cream, pour it in now and mix well.

When done, remove the soup from the heat and taste. Season it with more salt if needed. Remove the pepercorns and bay leaves before serving. Try with a dollop of sour cream and a side of Ultimate Keto Buns (page 24).

TIPS

- If you don't eat pork, you can use beef, such as braising steak, instead; however, beef may require additional cooking time.
- If you think the soup will be too sour for you, place the sauerkraut in a colander and rinse with cold water before adding it to the soup.
- Use a spice bag for easy removal of the peppercorns and bay leaf when the soup is done.

NUTRITION FACTS PER SERVING

Total carbs: 11.8 g	**Protein:** 17.7 g	**Macronutrient ratio:** Calories from carbs (9%), protein (21%), fat (70%)
Fiber: 4 g	**Fat:** 25.5 g	
Net carbs: 7.7 g	**Energy:** 345 kcal	

CREAM OF ZUCCHINI SOUP

Creamy and satisfying, this soup is the ultimate winter warmer, and it's extra-special when it's served with a dollop of sour cream or some crisp bacon.

6 SERVINGS	15 MINS	30 MINS

INGREDIENTS

2 large (500 g/17.6 oz) zucchini

1 large (200 g/7.1 oz) leek

2 tablespoons (30 g/1.1 oz) ghee or lard

2 cloves garlic, crushed

3 cups (720 ml/0.75 quart) chicken stock (page 128)

1 cup (240 ml/8 fl oz) heavy whipping cream or coconut milk

3 cups (375 g/13.1 oz) Simple Shredded Chicken (page 128)

Salt and freshly ground black pepper, to taste

2 tablespoons (8 g/0.3 oz) chopped fresh parsley or chives

Optional: 8 slices crisped bacon or 1 ½ cup (345 g/12 oz) sour cream on top

Wash and dice the zucchini and slice the leek. Soak the sliced leek in a bowl of water: any dirt will settle at the bottom of the bowl. Drain the leek well on a paper towel.

Heat the ghee in a large pot and add the crushed garlic. Cook for one minute and then add the zucchini and leek. Cook for about 5 minutes, stirring continuously.

Add the chicken stock and bring to a boil. Reduce the heat and simmer for about 20 minutes or until the leek and zucchini are tender. Remove from the heat.

Mix with a hand blender or pour into a food processor and pulse until smooth. Return the soup to the heat and add the heavy whipping cream and chicken. Cook for another 5 minutes to heat through. Season with salt and black pepper to taste. Garnish with chopped herbs. Try it with crisped-up bacon or sour cream on top and Ultimate Keto Buns (page 26) on the side.

NUTRITION FACTS PER SERVING

Total carbs: 8.8 g

Fiber: 1.5 g

Net carbs: 7.3 g

Protein: 16.4 g

Fat: 32.7 g

Energy: 393 kcal

Macronutrient ratio: Calories from carbs (7%), protein (17%), fat (76%)

CHICKEN MINESTRONE

My low-carb, paleo-friendly take on this traditional Italian soup is an easy way to make use of seasonal produce or frozen vegetables.

 8 SERVINGS | **20 MINS** | **50 MINS**

INGREDIENTS

1 medium (110 g/3.9 oz) white onion

2 cloves garlic, crushed

2 medium (80 g/2.8 oz) celery stalks

1 small (50 g/1.8 oz) leek

1 medium (200 g/7.1 oz) zucchini

1 ½ cups (150 g/5.3 oz) green beans

3 cups (210 g/7.4 oz) savoy cabbage, shredded

6 slices (90 g/3.2 oz) thinly-cut pancetta or bacon

2 tablespoons (30 g/1.1 oz) ghee or lard

2 bay leaves

3 cups (360 g/12.7 oz) diced canned tomatoes

2 quarts (2 liters/67.6 fl oz) chicken stock (page 128)

1 quart (1 liter/33.8 oz) water

4 cups (500 g/17.6 oz) Simple Shredded Chicken (page 128)

Salt and black pepper, to taste

Fresh basil and oregano to taste

½ cup (125 g/4.4 oz) pesto (page 35)

First, prepare the vegetables. Peel and slice the onion and crush the garlic. Wash and slice the celery stalks and leek. Wash and dice the zucchini. Wash, trim, and cut the green beans into thirds. Wash and shred or slice the savoy cabbage. Next, dice the pancetta.

Heat a large pot over a medium heat and add the ghee. Cook the onion and garlic just about 2 to 3 minutes before adding the sliced pancetta. Stir continuously until lightly browned.

Add the leek, zucchini, green beans, savoy cabbage, and bay leaf. Cook for about 10 minutes, stirring frequently. Add the tomatoes.

Pour in the chicken stock and bring to a boil. Cover with a lid and simmer for about 30 minutes or until the vegetables are tender. Add more water or stock if the soup is too thick. Season with salt and black pepper. Finally, add the Simply Shredded Chicken, basil, and oregano and remove from the heat.

Pour into bowls and finish each with a tablespoon (15 g/0.5 oz) of homemade pesto (or sprinkle with grated Parmesan cheese instead). Serve with Ultimate Keto Buns (page 26).

TIPS

· Try topping with a cup (100 g/3.5 oz) of Parmesan cheese instead of the pesto.
· This soup makes 8 servings, so if you're making it just for yourself, halve the recipe or freeze the remaining soup into manageable portions.

NUTRITION FACTS PER SERVING

Total carbs: 9.6 g	Protein: 18.9 g	Macronutrient ratio: Calories from carbs (7%), protein (21%), fat (72%)
Fiber: 3.2 g	Fat: 28.3 g	
Net carbs: 6.4 g	Energy: 371 kca	

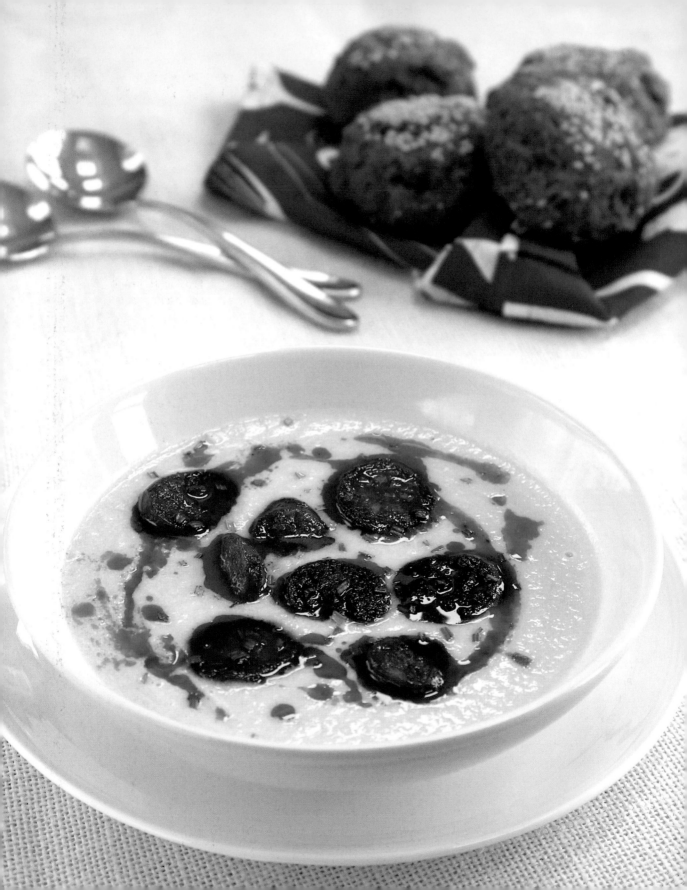

CREAMY CAULIFLOWER & CHORIZO SOUP

Hearty and warming, this sweet-and-spicy soup matches keto-friendly cauliflower with robust, meaty chorizo in a fantastic one-bowl meal.

 6 SERVINGS | **15 MINS** | **30 MINS**

INGREDIENTS

1 large (1 kg/2.2 lb) cauliflower

2 cloves garlic

1 medium (110 g/3.9 oz) white onion

3 tablespoons (45/1.6 oz) ghee or lard

Salt and freshly ground black pepper to taste

4 cups (about 1 liter/33.8 oz) chicken stock (page 128) or Bone Broth (page 30)

1 large (200 g/7.1 oz) Spanish chorizo

Leaves from 1 to 2 sprigs fresh rosemary, chopped

Optional: 1½ cup (336 g/12 oz) crème fraîche or heavy whipping cream

NUTRITION FACTS PER SERVING

Total carbs: 11 g

Fiber: 3.7 g

Net carbs: 7.3 g

Protein: 14.7 g

Fat: 24 g

Energy: 312 kcal

Macronutrient ratio: Calories from carbs (10%), protein (19%), fat (71%)

Wash the cauliflower and cut it into small florets. Peel and slice the garlic and onion. Heat 2 tablespoons (30 g/1.1 oz) of the ghee in a large pot and then sautée the onion and garlic over medium heat for about 10 minutes or until lightly browned, stirring frequently.

Add the cauliflower florets, salt, black pepper, and the chicken stock. Cover and simmer for about 15 minutes.

Meanwhile, finely slice or dice the chorizo and chop the rosemary. Heat the remaining ghee in a separate pan and add the chorizo and rosemary. Cook for about 5 minutes until the chorizo is crispy and set aside.

When the cauliflower is tender, remove the soup from the heat and set aside for 5 minutes. Blend with a hand blender to make the soup smooth and creamy or pour into a food processor and pulse. Ladle into serving bowls. Garnish each with the crisp chorizo and rosemary and drizzle in some of the chorizo juice.

SPICY THAI "NOODLE" SOUP

Use prawn shells to make your own fish stock in this quick and delicious soup infused with Asian flavors.

8 SERVINGS	20 MINS	1 HOUR

INGREDIENTS

1.3 pounds (600 g) prawns, shells on

Bunch fresh cilantro

3 tablespoons (45 g/1.6 oz) ghee or coconut oil

4 cloves garlic, crushed

1 medium (110 g/3.9 oz) white onion, peeled and diced

1 tablespoon (8 g/0.3 oz) ginger or galangal

1 lemongrass stalk, chopped

4 lime leaves or 2 teaspoons freshly grated lime zest

1 to 2 small hot chile peppers

2 quarts (2 liters/67.6 fl oz) chicken stock

½ pound (230 g) wild mushrooms, such as oyster

2 medium (400 g/14.1 oz) zucchini

1 small (300 g/10.6 oz) rutabaga

3 tablespoons (45 ml/1.5 fl oz) fish sauce

2 cups (480 ml/16 fl oz) coconut milk

Juice from 1 to 2 limes (about ¼ cup/60 ml/2 fl oz)

Salt and freshly ground black pepper, to taste

Peel and devein the prawns: reserve the shells for the fish stock. Meanwhile, store the raw prawns in the fridge. Wash and tear the cilantro leaves off the stalks; you'll use the stalks for the fish stock and the leaves for the final garnish. Wash, deseed, and finely chop the chile peppers.

Heat the ghee in a large pot over a medium heat and then add the prawn shells. Cook for a few minutes, stirring frequently, until the shells become red. Add the garlic, onion, ginger, lemongrass stalk, chopped cilantro stalks, lime leaves, and chopped chile peppers. Cook for about 5 minutes, continuing to stir frequently.

Pour the chicken stock into the pot and bring to a boil. Cover with a lid and simmer for about 30 minutes. When done, pour the broth through a sieve and discard any solids.

Clean and slice the mushrooms. Wash the zucchini and, using a julienne peeler or a vegetable spiralizer, peel the zucchini into thin "noodles." Alternatively, you can dice the zucchini into 1-inch pieces. Peel and dice the rutabaga into ½- to 1-inch (1.3 to 2.5 cm) pieces.

Return the broth to the heat. Add the mushrooms, zucchini, and rutabaga, followed by the fish sauce, coconut milk, lime juice, salt, and black pepper. Cook over medium heat for 15 to 20 minutes or until the rutabaga is tender. Add the raw prawns and cook for another 2 to 3 minutes. When done, spoon into serving dishes and garnish with the reserved cilantro leaves.

NUTRITION FACTS PER SERVING

Total carbs: 8.8 g	**Protein:** 15.8 g	**Macronutrient ratio:**
Fiber: 1.9 g	**Fat:** 22.2 g	Calories from carbs (9%), protein (22%), fat (69%)
Net carbs: 6.8 g	**Energy:** 284 kcal	

CREAMY KETO COLESLAW

Pair this addictive salad with roasted meats or use it as a filling in low-carb buns.

4 SERVINGS	10 MINS	10 MINS

INGREDIENTS

½ head (400 g/14.1 oz) green or white cabbage

1 small (50 g/1.8 oz) carrot

1 small (60 g/2.1 oz) red onion

¼ cup (55 g/1.9 oz) Mayonnaise (page 28)

¼ cup (60 g/2.1 oz) sour cream or more mayonnaise

1 tablespoon (15 ml/0.5 fl oz) lemon juice

1 tablespoon (15 ml/0.5 fl oz) apple cider vinegar

½ teaspoon celery seeds

1 teaspoon Dijon (page 31) or wholegrain mustard

Salt and freshly ground black pepper to taste

Optional: 1 tablespoon (10 g/ 0.4 oz) erythritol or Swerve or 5 drops liquid stevia

Wash and cut the cabbage in half. Remove the hard stem and, using either a sharp knife or a mandolin, finely slice the cabbage. Place in a bowl. Peel and julienne the carrot and thinly slice the red onion. Add to the bowl with the cabbage.

For the dressing, in a mixing bowl, combine the mayonnaise, sour cream, lemon juice, apple cider vinegar, celery seeds, and whole grain mustard. Season with salt and black pepper to taste. Add the dressing to the bowl with the vegetables and toss well. Serve immediately or store in an airtight container for up to 3 days.

TIP

Go ahead and make your coleslaw in advance and then store it in the fridge for an hour or two: it tastes best if you let the flavors combine for a little while before serving.

NUTRITION FACTS PER SERVING

Total carbs: 9.3 g	**Protein:** 2 g	**Macronutrient ratio:** Calories from carbs (15%), protein (5%), fat (80%)
Fiber: 3.2 g	**Fat:** 14.8 g	
Net carbs: 6.1 g	**Energy:** 167 kcal	

VEGETARIAN STUFFED AVOCADO

Some days you just don't feel like eating meat—and that's when you'll reach for this light, bright combination of avocado, sweet celeriac, and lemon.

 2 SERVINGS | **10 MINS** | **5 MINS**

INGREDIENTS

1 small (120 g/4.2 oz) celeriac

2 large (400 g/14.1 oz) avocados, halved

2 tablespoons (30 ml/1 fl oz) freshly squeezed lemon juice

2 teaspoons freshly grated lemon zest

4 tablespoons (60 g/2.1 oz) Mayonnaise (page 28)

Salt and freshly ground black pepper to taste

NUTRITION FACTS PER SERVING

Total carbs: 23.8 g

Fiber: 14.9 g

Net carbs: 8.9 g

Protein: 5.6 g

Fat: 54.3 g

Energy: 570 kcal

Macronutrient ratio: Calories from carbs (7%), protein (4%), fat (89%)

Peel the celeriac. Using a grater with the smallest holes, finely grate the celeriac into a bowl. Leaving a ¼- to ½-inch (6 to 13 mm) layer of avocado along the insides of the skins, scoop the middle of the avocado halves out into a bowl with the celeriac. Add the lemon juice, lemon zest, mayonnaise, salt, and black pepper and combine. Fill the avocado halves with the mixture and enjoy!

TIP

Instead of mayo, you can substitute the same amount of cream cheese or healthy oils, such as avocado, macadamia, or extra virgin olive oil.

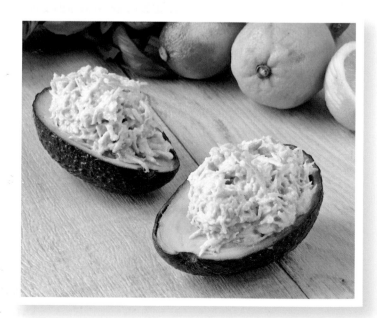

GRATED GREEN & FETA SALAD

This Greek-style salad makes a super summertime lunch or dinner.
And it's even better when it's topped with crispy bacon!

4 SERVINGS	5 MINS	5 MINS

INGREDIENTS

1 large (300 g/10.6 oz) cucumber

1 large (300 g/10.6 oz) zucchini

1 large (150 g/5.3 oz) green pepper

2 medium (30 g/1.1 oz) spring onions

2 cups (300 g/10.6 oz) feta cheese, crumbled

Dressing

3 tablespoons (45 ml/1.5 fl oz) extra virgin olive oil

2 tablespoons (30 ml/1 fl oz) freshly squeezed lemon juice

2 tablespoons (12 g/0.4 oz) chopped fresh mint

¼ teaspoon chile flakes

Salt and freshly ground black pepper, to taste

NUTRITION FACTS PER SERVING

Total carbs: 10.2 g

Fiber: 2.3 g

Net carbs: 7.8 g

Protein: 12.6 g

Fat: 26.6 g

Energy: 322 kcal

Macronutrient ratio: Calories from carbs (10%), protein (16%), fat (74%)

Wash and grate the cucumber and zucchini. You can use a julienne peeler or a spiralizer to slice them and create thin "noodles." Wash, deseed, and thinly slice the green bell pepper. Wash and slice the spring onions. Add the feta cheese.

To make the dressing, mix together all the ingredients. Pour it over the salad and combine well. Let it sit for 5 to 10 minutes before serving. Top with crispy bacon, if you like.

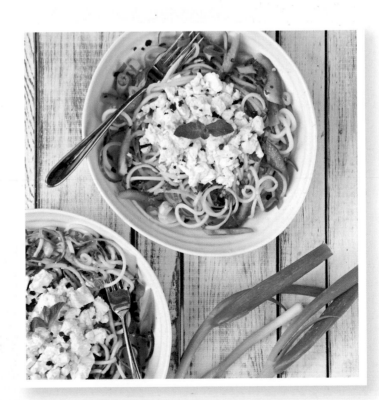

CAESAR SALAD IN A CHEESE BOWL

Use your favorite cheese to make these fun bowls—then pack them
with Caesar salad for a luscious low-carb lunch.

2 SERVINGS	20 MINS	30 MINS

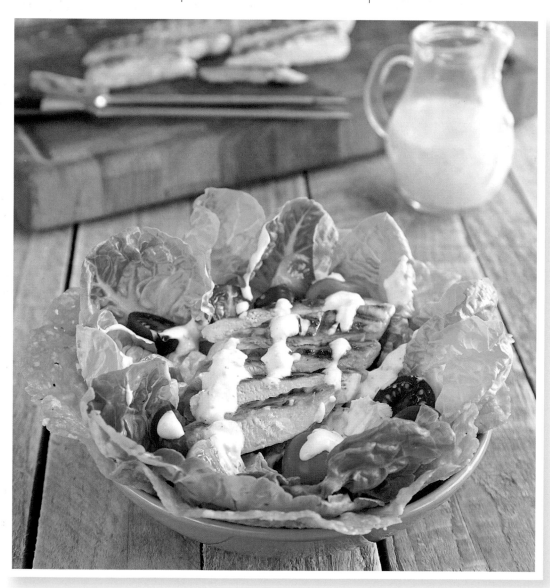

INGREDIENTS
Caesar Salad
1½ cups (150 g/5.3 oz) grated Parmesan cheese

4 slices (60 g/2.1 oz) thinly-cut bacon

2 small (200 g/7.1 oz) chicken breasts

1 tablespoon (15 g/0.5 oz) ghee or coconut oil

Salt and freshly ground black pepper, to taste

2 small (200 g/7.1 oz) heads lettuce

1 cup (150 g/5.3 oz) cherry tomatoes

Dressing
3 tablespoons (36 g/1.3 oz) sour cream or Mayonnaise (page 28)

1 tablespoon (15 ml/0.5 fl oz) extra virgin olive oil

1 clove garlic, crushed

2 tablespoons (30 ml/1 fl oz) freshly squeezed lemon juice

1 teaspoon Dijon Mustard (page 31)

2 teaspoons oregano, dried

Salt and freshly ground black pepper to taste

NUTRITION FACTS PER SERVING
Total carbs: 10.5 g

Fiber: 2.9 g

Net carbs: 7.6 g

Protein: 53.3 g

Fat: 45.3 g

Energy: 663 kcal

Macronutrient ratio: Calories from carbs (5%), protein (33%), fat (62%)

First, prepare the cheese bowl. Preheat the oven to 400°F (200°C, or gas mark 6) and line a baking sheet with parchment paper cut in half (one half per cheese bowl). Grate the Parmesan cheese and spread on the baking sheet into in the shape of two rough circles. The Parmesan cheese won't melt as much as other types of cheese with higher fat contents, like cheddar, so the size of the cheese circle will be almost the same after it's baked. Keep that in mind when arranging the cheese, since you'll need to be able to create a cheese "bowl" from it.

Bake in the oven for about 5 minutes. Watch it carefully: The cheese crust should be golden in color, not brown. If you bake it for too long, it will taste bitter. When done, remove from the oven and allow to cool for about a minute.

To create the cheese bowl, set a small bowl upside-down and then carefully lift the parchment paper off the tray and flip the cheese over the bowl. Lightly press the edges, if needed, and let cool in that position for at least 5 minutes. You can leave the cheese on the bowl while you prepare the salad filling.

Pan-fry the bacon strips until crisp. When done, tear or slice the bacon into smaller pieces. Brush the chicken breast with ghee and season with salt and black pepper to taste. Cook on a griddle pan or a regular pan on both sides until the top is brown and crispy and the inside is cooked through. When done, let the chicken cool slightly on a cutting board before slicing into strips.

Prepare the dressing by mixing the sour cream or mayo, olive oil, crushed garlic clove, lemon juice, Dijon mustard, and oregano. Season with salt and black pepper and set aside.

Wash and pat dry the lettuce leaves and arrange them in the cheese bowl. Wash and slice the cherry tomatoes. Add the cherry tomatoes, sliced bacon, and chicken strips. Pour the dressing over top. Enjoy while the chicken is still warm.

TIPS
- If you find that making the cheese bowls is too challenging, make small cheese crisps instead and serve alongside the salad. Simply scoop a teaspoon of the grated cheese onto a baking sheet lined with parchment paper and repeat until you use up all the cheese, leaving a small gap between each. Bake for 10 to 15 minutes or until crispy.
- You can try making cheese bowls with other types of cheese such as Cheddar or gouda.

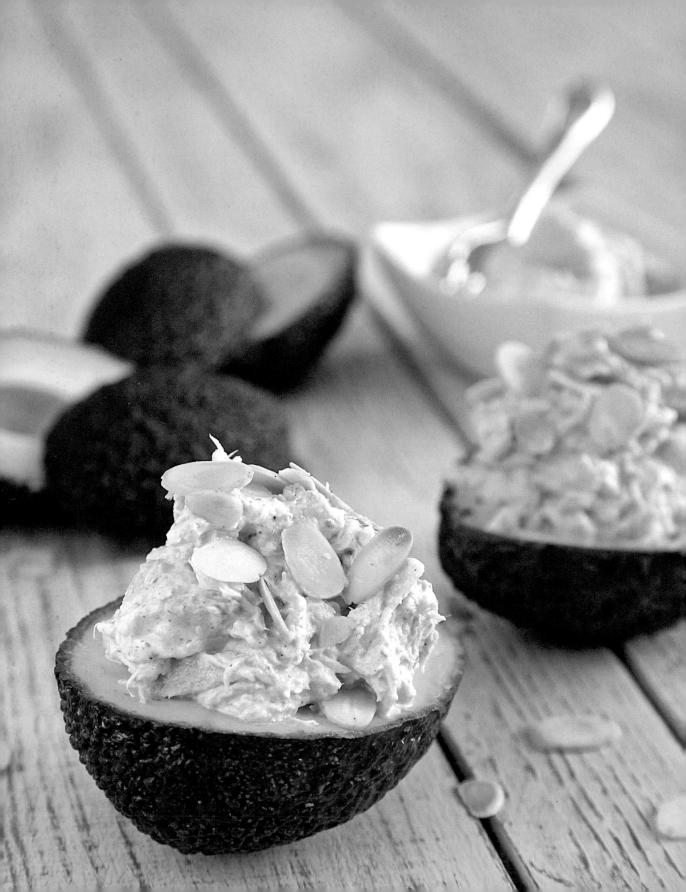

CURRIED CHICKEN STUFFED AVOCADO

There's practically zero work involved in whipping up this light lunch, as long as you have a batch of Simple Shredded Chicken (page 128) on hand.

2 SERVINGS	5 MINS	5 MINS

INGREDIENTS

Avocado Boats

2 medium (300 g/10.6 oz) avocados

2 cups (250 g/8.8 oz) Simple Shredded Chicken (page 128)

2 tablespoons (10 g/0.4 oz) flaked almonds, toasted

Dressing

¼ cup (58 g/2 oz) sour cream or Mayonnaise (page 28)

¼ teaspoon ground turmeric

¼ teaspoon ground ginger

½ teaspoon curry powder

1 clove garlic, crushed

Salt and freshly ground black pepper, to taste

NUTRITION FACTS PER SERVING

Total carbs: 15.7 g

Fiber: 2.3 g

Net carbs: 4.8 g

Protein: 28.3 g

Fat: 50.1 g

Energy: 601 kcal

Macronutrient ratio: Calories from carbs (3%), protein (20%), fat (77%)

Make the dressing by mixing together all the ingredients and then set aside.

Halve the avocado and remove the pit. Leaving about ½ to 1 inch (1.3 to 2.5 cm) of the avocado flesh in the skin, scoop out the middle of the avocado.

Place the avocado flesh, Simple Shredded Chicken, dressing, and toasted almonds in a bowl and combine well. Leave a few almond slices aside for garnish.

Finally, top each avocado half with the mixture and garnish with the remaining toasted almonds.

TIPS

- This salad is best eaten immediately. If you're taking it to work, don't cut the avocado beforehand; this will prevent it from browning. Add the filling to it just before eating.

- Toasting sliced almonds is easy: just dry-fry them in a pan for a minute or two. Make sure you don't burn them or they'll taste bitter.

COBB SALAD IN A "TORTILLA" BOWL

Nothing will keep you fuller for longer than this bacon-and-blue-cheese-laden Cobb salad, served in a delicious low-carb tortilla bowl!

2 SERVINGS	15 MINS	20 MINS

INGREDIENTS

Cobb Salad

2 Grain-free Tortilla Bowls (medium-size, about 8 inches/20 cm) (page 25)

2 large eggs

2 slices (50 g/1.8 oz) ham

2 slices (30 g/1.1 oz) of thinly-cut bacon

½ cup (75 g/2.6 oz) cherry tomatoes

1 cup (30 g/1.1 oz) watercress

2 small (200 g/7.1 oz) heads of lettuce

1 medium (150 g/5.3 oz) avocado

⅓ cup (50 g/1.8 oz) blue cheese, crumbled

1 cup (125 g/4.4 oz) Simple Shredded Chicken (page 128)

Dressing

2 tablespoons (30 ml/1 fl oz) extra virgin olive oil

1 teaspoon each red wine vinegar, Dijon Mustard (page 31), and Worcestershire sauce

1 tablespoon (15 ml/0.5 fl oz) lemon juice

1 clove garlic, crushed

Salt and freshly ground black pepper, to taste

Prepare the tortilla bowl by following the recipe in Grain-free Tortillas. Hard boil the eggs.

Slice the ham and bacon and crisp them up in a pan. Lightly grease the pan if needed.

Wash and slice the tomatoes. Wash the watercress and lettuce and tear the lettuce into smaller pieces. Dry well in a salad spinner or by patting with a paper towel. Peel the eggs and slice or quarter them with a knife. Peel, deseed, and slice the avocado. Prepare the dressing by mixing all the ingredients and set aside.

Assemble the salad. Start by placing the lettuce, watercress, and sliced tomatoes in a salad bowl. Top with the tortilla bowl. Fill the tortilla bowl with the bacon, ham, avocado, sliced egg, crumbled blue cheese, and Simple Shredded Chicken. Drizzle both the lettuce and the tortilla filling with the prepared dressing and serve immediately; if left for too long, the tortilla will become soggy.

TIPS

- To make this a work-friendly lunch, pack everything apart from the tortilla in an airtight container. Make a regular tortilla or create crispy "nachos" and store in a separate container to serve with the salad.

- For a sweeter dressing, add 1 tablespoon (10 g/0.4 oz) of erythritol or Swerve, or 3 to 5 drops of liquid stevia.

NUTRITION FACTS PER SERVING

Total carbs: 20.4 g **Protein:** 37.4 g **Macronutrient ratio:**
Fiber: 12.4 g **Fat:** 65.5 g Calories from carbs (4%), protein (19%),
Net carbs: 8 g **Energy:** 797 kcal fat (77%)

Chapter Seven:

MAIN MEALS

Sustaining any diet or eating plan on a long-term basis often boils down to knowing what to put on the dinner table every night. The evening meal traditionally contains the highest amount of protein, since meat, poultry, or fish often features as the main course—and the good news is, these foods are totally keto-friendly. Just be sure to prepare them with ingredients that are high in healthy fats, such as ghee, olive oil, homemade mayonnaise, avocados, or nuts. Always remember to opt for pastured poultry, grass-fed meat, and sustainable, wild-caught fish as much as your budget will allow.

PALEO CHICKEN NUGGETS

You'll love this healthy alternative
to the popular take-away meal.

 4 SERVINGS | **15 MINS** | **30 MINS**

INGREDIENTS

1½ pounds (680 g) chicken breast, skinless and boneless

½ teaspoon salt

1 large egg

1 tablespoon (15 ml/0.5 fl oz) almond milk or coconut milk

1 cup (100 g/3.5 oz) almond flour

1 teaspoon paprika

1 teaspoon onion powder

1 teaspoon garlic powder

⅓ cup (30 g/1.1 oz) grated Parmesan cheese or more almond flour

2 tablespoons (30 g/1 oz) coconut oil or ghee

Optional: ¼ cup (65 g/2.3 oz) Spicy Chocolate BBQ Sauce (page 34), Ketchup (page 29), Dijon Mustard (page 31) or Mayonnaise (page 28), to serve

Preheat the oven to 400°F (200°C, or gas mark 6). Using a paper towel, dab any excess moisture from the chicken. Dice the chicken breasts into medium-sized pieces and season with half of the salt.

Mix the egg with the almond milk and season with the rest of the salt. Place the chicken pieces into the egg mixture.

Mix the dry ingredients (the almond flour through the grated Parmesan cheese) and pour into a large baking sheet.

Lift up each piece of chicken, let some of the egg mixture drip off, and then transfer to the baking sheet. (Avoid dribbling in any excess egg mixture or else it will clump up the dry ingredients.) Cover all sides of the chicken pieces with the dry mixture. Do this in batches and do not overfill the baking sheet.

Move the coated chicken nuggets to a baking sheet lined with parchment paper, drizzle with ghee, and transfer to the oven. Cook for about 15 minutes until lightly golden. Remove the tray from the oven and let cool for a few minutes. Serve with Spicy Chocolate BBQ Sauce, Mayonnaise, Ketchup, or Dijon Mustard.

TIP

For a nut-free alternative, try powdered pork rinds instead of almond flour.

NUTRITION FACTS PER SERVING

Total carbs: 6.3 g | **Protein:** 46 g | **Macronutrient ratio:**
Fiber: 2.8 g | **Fat:** 28.3 g | Calories from carbs (3%), protein (41%), fat (56%)
Net carbs: 3.5 g | **Energy:** 463 kcal |

CHICKEN SATAY WITH "PEANUT" SAUCE

I've adjusted this popular Asian dish to suit a paleo, keto-friendly diet— and I think it's even better than the traditional take-out version!

4 SERVINGS	15 MINS	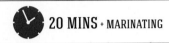 20 MINS + MARINATING

INGREDIENTS

Chicken

1.3 pounds (600 g) chicken thighs

2 tablespoons (30 ml/1 fl oz) each coconut aminos, lemon juice and coconut oil

2 cloves garlic, crushed

¼ teaspoon salt

2 medium (30 g/1.1 oz) spring onions or chives

Satay Sauce

½ cup (130 g/4.6 oz) Toasted Coconut Butter (page 39) or almond butter

½ cup (120 ml/4 fl oz) coconut milk or heavy whipping cream

1 tablespoon (15 ml/0.5 fl oz) each coconut aminos, fish sauce and lemon juice

2 teaspoons freshly grated ginger

1 clove garlic, crushed

¼ teaspoon salt

Dice the chicken thigh meat and place it in a bowl with the coconut aminos, lemon juice, and crushed garlic and season with salt. Marinate in the fridge for at least 1 hour or overnight.

Meanwhile, prepare the satay sauce. Put all the ingredients in a bowl and mix until well combined.

Preheat the oven to 475°F (245°C, or gas mark 9) or, ideally, broil (500°F [260°C, or gas mark 10]). Remove the chicken from the fridge and pierce onto skewers. Drizzle each skewer with coconut oil, turning to coat on all sides, and place on a rack on top of a baking sheet. Transfer to the oven and cook for about 10 minutes. Turn the skewers over halfway through the cooking process.

Remove the chicken from the oven and let it cool before transferring to a serving plate. Garnish with chopped spring onion and serve with the prepared satay sauce.

NUTRITION FACTS PER SERVING

Total carbs: 9.8 g   **Protein:** 34.1 g

Fiber: 3.9 g   **Fat:** 39.6 g

Net carbs: 5.8 g   **Energy:** 515 kcal

Macronutrient ratio: Calories from carbs (5%), protein (26%), fat (69%)

SPATCHCOCK BBQ CHICKEN

There's no better way to cook chicken than to spatchcock it.
It's ready in a fraction of the time it takes to roast a chicken,
and it's crispy on the outside but so juicy on the inside.

 4 SERVINGS | 10 MINS | 50 TO 60 MINS

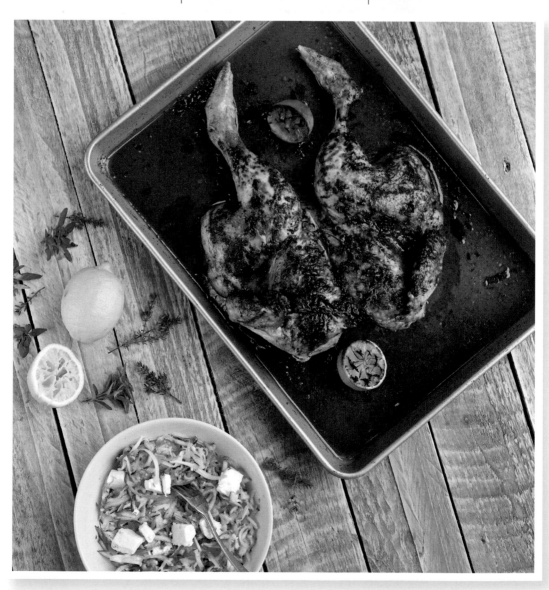

INGREDIENTS

1 whole chicken (about 1.4 kg/ 3 lb, bones included)

2 tablespoons (5 g/0.2 oz) chopped fresh herbs or 2 teaspoons dried (oregano, basil, thyme)

1 tablespoon (7 g/0.3 oz) paprika

1 teaspoon onion powder

1 teaspoon garlic powder

¼ teaspoon chile powder

¼ teaspoon freshly ground black pepper

1 teaspoon salt

1 lemon, halved and juiced

2 tablespoons (30 g/1.1 oz) ghee or butter

½ cup (120 ml/4 fl oz) chicken stock or Bone Broth (page 30)

NUTRITION FACTS PER SERVING

Total carbs: 3.3 g

Fiber: 1.1 g

Net carbs: 2.2 g

Protein: 29.1 g

Fat: 31.8 g

Energy: 412 kcal

Macronutrient ratio: Calories from carbs (2%), protein (28%), fat (70%)

Preheat the oven to 400°F (200°C, or gas mark 6). Remove the chicken from the fridge and let it sit on the kitchen counter while you prepare the seasoning.

To make the seasoning, wash and chop the herbs, if using fresh herbs. Mix with the paprika, onion powder, garlic powder, chile powder, black pepper, and salt.

Put the chicken on a cutting board, breast-side down. Using kitchen scissors, start snipping the chicken where its backbone cuts down from the tail along each side. Keep the backbone to make chicken stock (page 128) or Bone Broth (page 30).

Open the chicken and cut the cartilage covering the breastbone using a sharp knife. Rub some of the seasoning and lemon juice inside the chicken. Flip the chicken over and press down to flatten it.

Using your fingers, rub the ghee or butter under the skin. To do this, simply pull up the skin of the chicken and massage the fat into the flesh. Spread the remaining ghee on top of the skin: this will help the skin become crispy. Rub the chicken with the rest of the seasoning and squeeze the remaining lemon juice all over.

Push the tips of the wings behind the breastbone where the neck is. Place the chicken cut-side down in a baking sheet. Place the lemon halves on the sheet and pour in the chicken stock. Cook in the oven for 45 to 50 minutes. Baste the juices over the chicken once or twice during the cooking process.

The chicken is done when a meat thermometer in the breast meat reaches 150°F (65°C) and the thighs 170°F (77°C). Remove from the oven and let rest for 10 to 15 minutes before cutting it in quarters. Try it with Grated Green & Feta Salad (page 107).

TIP

For even crispier chicken, line a rimmed baking sheet with parchment paper or aluminum foil. Place a roasting rack on the tray, top with the chicken, and bake. The rack keeps the chicken above the baking sheet so air can circulate under it as it cooks.

CHICKEN KIEV

Rich and decadent—but keto-friendly!—this is the last word in comfort food. As always, seek out the best ingredients: pastured chicken breast, grass-fed butter, and pastured bacon.

 4 SERVINGS | **20 MINS** | **1 HOUR 30 MINS**

INGREDIENTS

Chicken

4 slices (60 g/2.1 oz) of thinly-cut bacon

1 large egg

4 medium (480 g/16.9 oz) chicken breasts

2 tablespoons (30 g/1.1 oz) ghee or coconut oil

Breading

¼ cup plus 1 tablespoon (35 g/1.3 oz) almond flour

¼ cup plus 1 tablespoon (50 g/1.8 oz) flax meal

⅓ cup (30 g/1.1 oz) grated Parmesan cheese or more almond flour

Pinch salt

Herb Butter

¼ cup (56 g/2 oz) butter or ghee, softened to room temperature

2 tablespoons (8 g/0.3 oz) chopped fresh parsley

2 tablespoons (5 g/02. oz) chopped fresh basil

2 cloves garlic, crushed

Salt and freshly ground black pepper to taste

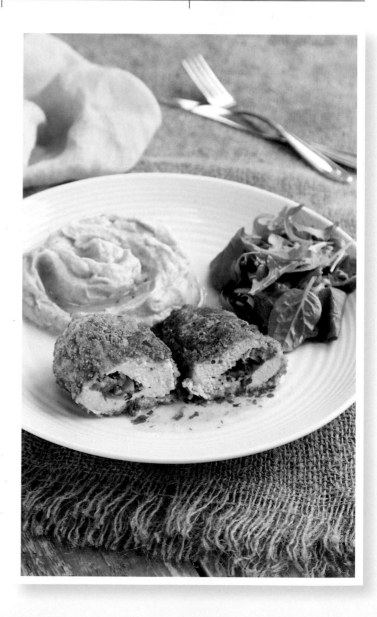

NUTRITION FACTS PER SERVING

Total carbs: 5.8 g

Fiber: 4 g

Net carbs: 1.8 g

Protein: 36 g

Fat: 38.3 g

Energy: 510 kcal

Macronutrient ratio:
Calories from carbs (1%),
protein (29%), fat (70%)

Prepare the herb butter. Mix the softened butter with the chopped herbs and crushed garlic. Season with the salt and black pepper and place on parchment paper. Roll the paper around the butter to shape it and then tighten and twist the ends of the parchment. Place in the fridge to firm up for about an hour.

Fry the bacon in a pan greased with 1 tablespoon (15 g/0.5 oz) of the ghee until crisp. Transfer to a plate to cool and then crumble or cut into small pieces.

Prepare the breading by mixing the almond flour, flax meal, and Parmesan on a large plate. Season with salt.

Crack the egg into a separate bowl and then whisk it and season with salt.

When the butter is chilled and firm, stuff the chicken breast. Set the chicken breast on a cutting board and use a sharp knife to cut the thickest part of it, creating a long pocket. Angle your slice diagonally, rather than horizontally, to prevent too much of the filling from leaking out. Don't cut the breast all the way through or the butter will seep out when heated.

Slice the herb butter into small pieces. Squeeze a slice of butter into the pocket you've cut in the chicken. Add some crumbled bacon and squeeze in more herb butter. Fold and seal the pocket tightly. Repeat for all the chicken breasts.

Preheat the oven to 350°F (175°C, or gas mark 4). Dip each chicken breast in the egg and let any excess drip off before dredging the chicken in the breading. Evenly coat the chicken on all sides. Set aside.

Add another tablespoon (15 g/0.5 oz) of the ghee to the pan in which you cooked the bacon and set to a medium-high heat. Once the pan is hot, fry each chicken breast for 2 to 3 minutes per side. Work in batches as needed. To keep the breading from getting stuck to the pan, make sure the pan is really hot. Avoid turning the chicken too soon and do not turn more than once to keep the breading from falling off.

Gently transfer the breasts into a baking dish and cook in the in the oven for 10 minutes. When done, remove the chicken from the oven and set on a cooling rack for a few minutes.

BUFFALO CHICKEN WINGS
WITH RANCH DRESSING

These crispy chicken wings are a healthy version of the popular bar snack. Make them into a meal by serving them with freshly-cut vegetables or Creamy Keto Coleslaw (page 105).

 4 SERVINGS | **10 MINS** | 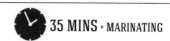 **35 MINS** + MARINATING

INGREDIENTS

¼ cup (60 g/2.1 oz) Spicy Chocolate BBQ Sauce (page 34)

1 tablespoon (15 ml/0.5 fl oz) extra virgin olive oil

5 pounds (2.3 kg, approximately 20 to 24 pieces) chicken wings

1 tablespoon (7 g/0.25 oz) paprika

1 teaspoon each onion powder and garlic powder

½ teaspoon salt

Freshly ground black pepper

2 tablespoons (30 g/1.1 oz) ghee or coconut oil

Ranch Dressing

¼ cup (60 g/2.1 oz) sour cream or creamed coconut milk

¼ cup (60 ml/2 fl oz) heavy whipping cream or more coconut milk

½ cup (110g/3.9 oz) Mayonnaise (page 28)

2 medium spring onions or chives (30 g/1.1 oz)

1 clove garlic, crushed

2 tablespoons (8 g/0.3 oz) chopped fresh parsley

1 tablespoon (4 g/0.1 oz) chopped fresh dill

(continued)

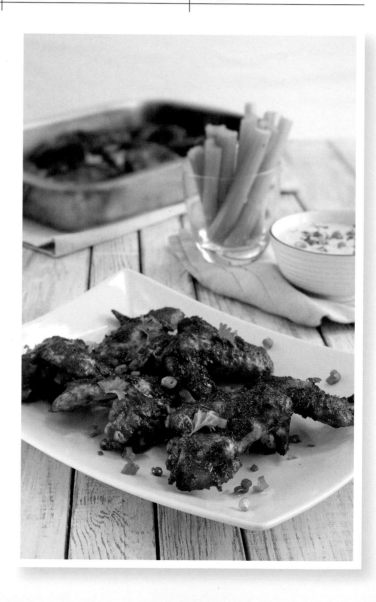

1 tablespoon (15 ml/0.5 fl oz) apple cider vinegar

¼ teaspoon paprika

Salt and freshly ground black pepper, to taste

NUTRITION FACTS PER SERVING

(5 to 6 wings)

Total carbs: 5.4 g

Fiber: 1.6 g

Net carbs: 3.8 g

Protein: 28.5 g

Fat: 59.4 g

Energy: 669 kcal

Macronutrient ratio:
Calories from carbs (2%), protein (17%), fat (81%)

Mix the Spicy Chocolate BBQ Sauce with the olive oil and then rub the mixture all over the chicken wings. Let the wings marinate in the fridge for at least an hour or overnight: the longer you marinate the wings, the more flavorful they'll be.

Once the chicken has had time to marinate, remove the wings from the fridge. Mix the paprika, onion and garlic powder, salt, and black pepper in a small bowl.

Preheat the oven to 400°F (200°C, or gas mark 6) and line a baking sheet with parchment paper. Place the chicken wings on a cutting board and discard any remaining marinade left in the bowl. Sprinkle the spice mix on all sides of the chicken.

Heat a large pan greased with ghee over a medium-high heat. When hot, add the chicken wings. Working in batches of four, fry the wings quickly on both sides, just for half a minute, and then place on the baking sheet. This will help the wings crisp up and will enhance the flavor.

When all the wings are ready, transfer the tray to the oven and bake for 20 to 25 minutes. Keep an eye on them to prevent burning. Meanwhile, prepare the ranch dressing. Mix all the ingredients in a small bowl and set aside. When the wings have cooked through, remove the tray from the oven. Serve the wings with the ranch dressing.

TIP

There are several options for dairy-free substitutes when making ranch dressing. Try smooth nut or coconut butter, mayonnaise, coconut milk, or almond milk. If the dressing isn't thick enough, add a tablespoon (13 g/0.5 oz) of ground chia seeds and set aside for 5 to 10 minutes. If the dressing is too thick, add some almond or coconut milk or water.

CRISPY BBQ CHICKEN DRUMSTICKS

These "breaded" drumsticks taste so much better than their
fast-food counterparts! Serve them with Zucchini Fries (page 193)
or Creamy Keto Coleslaw (page 105).

 5 SERVINGS | 15 MINS | 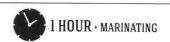 1 HOUR + MARINATING

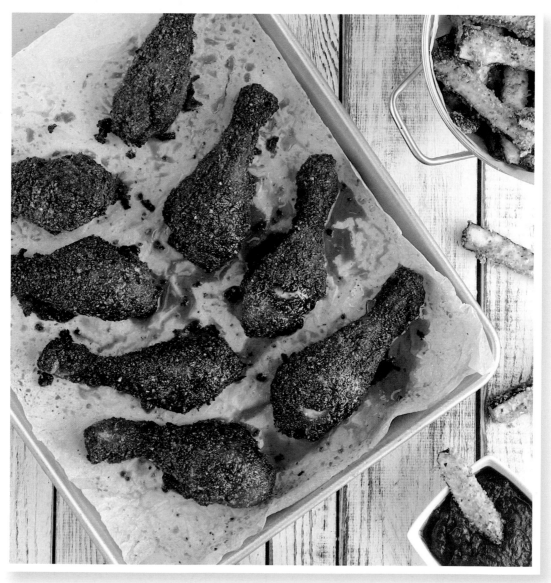

INGREDIENTS
Chicken Drumsticks
¼ cup (60 g/2.1 oz) Spicy Chocolate BBQ Sauce (page 34)

1 tablespoon (15 ml/0.5 fl oz) extra virgin olive oil

2.6 pounds (1.2 kg, approx. 10 pieces) chicken drumsticks

Breading
¾ cup (75 g/2.6 oz) almond flour or 1 cup (50 g/1.8 oz) ground pork rinds

¼ cup (40 g/1.4 oz) flax meal

1 teaspoon paprika

1 teaspoon garlic powder

1 teaspoon onion powder

½ teaspoon baking soda

1 teaspoon cream of tartar

¼ teaspoon salt

Freshly ground black pepper, to taste

2 tablespoons (30 g/1.1 oz) ghee or coconut oil

NUTRITION FACTS PER SERVING
(2 drumsticks)

Total carbs: 7.8 g

Fiber: 4.3 g

Net carbs: 3.5 g

Protein: 28 g

Fat: 33.3 g

Energy: 438 kcal

Macronutrient ratio:
Calories from carbs (3%), protein (26%), fat (71%)

Mix the Spicy Chocolate BBQ Sauce with the olive oil. Set the chicken drumsticks into a large dish and pour the sauce-and-oil mixture over top. Let the drumsticks marinate in the fridge for at least an hour or as long as overnight.

Preheat the oven to 350°F (175°C, or gas mark 4). Meanwhile, prepare the breading by mixing together the almond flour, flax meal, paprika, garlic powder, onion powder, baking soda, cream of tartar, salt, and black pepper.

Dredge each drumstick in the breading and then set on a baking sheet lined with parchment paper. The BBQ sauce acts as "glue" that the breading sticks to. Do not place all the chicken in the breading at once or it will clump up. Spray or drizzle the breaded drumsticks with melted ghee and then bake in the oven for 45 to 50 minutes.

When done, remove from the oven and serve immediately or refrigerate and reheat later, if needed. If the breading gets soggy, simply bake the chicken in the oven for another 5 minutes to crisp up before serving.

TIPS
- You can use all sorts of ingredients to make low-carb "breading." Mix your favorite spices and dried herbs with almond flour, coconut flour, flax meal, ground pork rinds, or grated Parmesan cheese.

- You can substitute 2 teaspoons of gluten-free baking powder for the baking soda and cream of tartar.

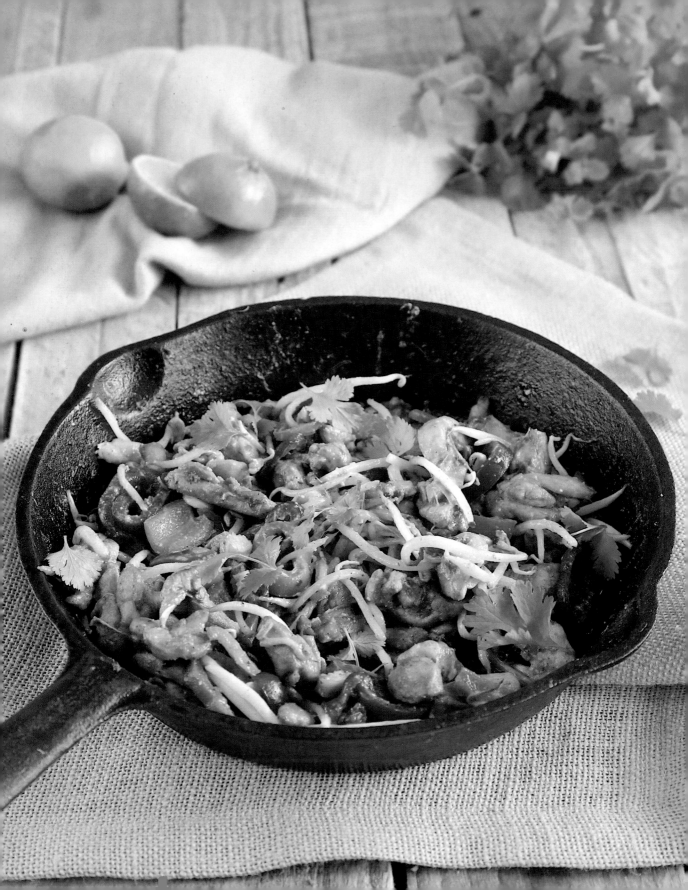

THAI-STYLE CHICKEN STIR-FRY

This easy chicken dish can be made ahead in just a few minutes—
perfect for days when you have no time to cook!

 4 SERVINGS | **15 MINS** | **20 MINS** + MARINATING

INGREDIENTS

1 pound (450 g) chicken thighs, skin and bones removed

2 tablespoons (30 ml/1.0 fl oz) fish sauce

1 tablespoon (15 ml/0.5 fl oz) coconut aminos

2 (300 g/10.6 oz) sweet bell peppers, red, orange or yellow

2 medium (30 g/1.1 oz) spring onions

1 tablespoon (8 g/0.3 oz) freshly grated ginger

2 cloves garlic

1 small hot chile pepper

¼ cup (56 g/2 oz) ghee or coconut oil

2 cups (100 g/3.5 oz) bean sprouts

¼ cup (65 g/2.3 oz) Toasted Nut Butter (page 39)

1 tablespoon (15 ml/0.5 fl oz) lime juice

Salt and black pepper to taste

2 tablespoons (2 g/0.07 oz) fresh cilantro

Slice the chicken thighs into medium pieces and add the fish sauce and coconut aminos. Marinate in the fridge for at least an hour or overnight.

Meanwhile, prepare the vegetables: Wash and slice the bell peppers and spring onions. Peel and grate the ginger and crush the garlic. Wash, deseed, and dice the chile pepper.

Place half of the ghee in a large pan and heat over medium-high heat. Add the chicken to the hot pan and keep stirring until the chicken is cooked and all the sides are browned. Remove the chicken from the pan and set aside in a bowl.

Grease the pan with the remaining ghee; add the ginger, garlic, and chile pepper. Cook for 2 to 3 minutes over medium-high heat, stirring frequently. Add the sliced bell pepper and spring onion and then season with salt and black pepper. Cook for another 5 minutes and add the bean sprouts.

Cook for one more minute. Finally, add the chicken, Toasted Nut Butter, and lime juice and combine well. Cook until the chicken is heated through. Garnish with fresh cilantro and season with more salt if needed.

NUTRITION FACTS PER SERVING

Total carbs: 11.3 g   **Protein:** 25.9 g   **Macronutrient ratio:** Calories from carbs (7%), protein (27%), fat (66%)

Fiber: 4.2 g   **Fat:** 28.9 g

Net carbs: 7.1 g   **Energy:** 405 kcal

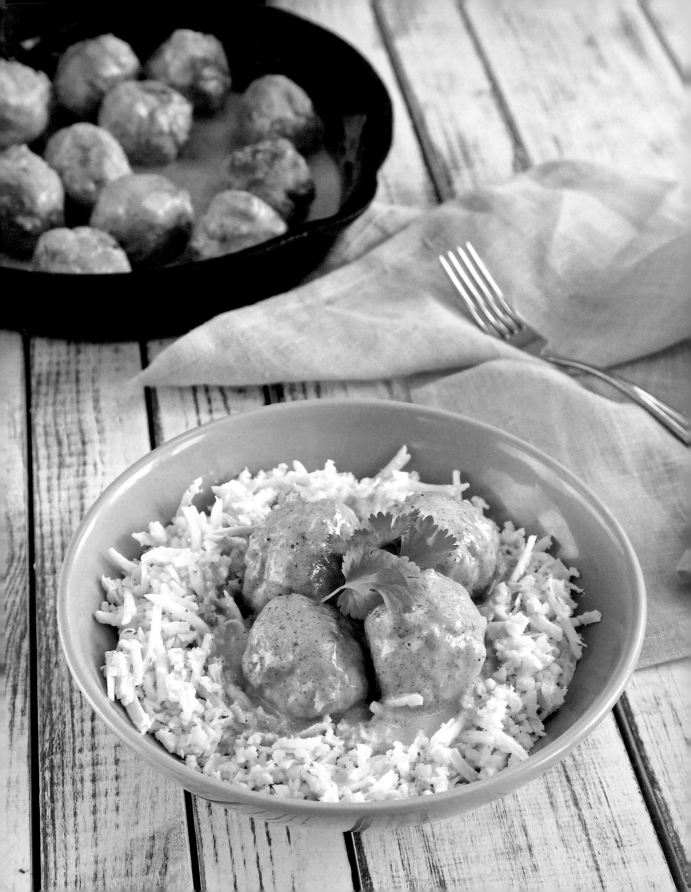

CHICKEN CURRY MEATBALLS

Healthy and quick to prepare, this meal combines two of my all-time favorites: meatballs and chicken curry.

16 MEATBALLS	15 MINS	20 MINS

INGREDIENTS

1.1 pounds (500 g) ground chicken

¼ cup (30 g/1.1 oz) coconut flour

1 large egg

2 cloves garlic, crushed

½ teaspoon ground turmeric

2 teaspoons curry powder

Salt to taste

2 tablespoons (30 g/1.1 oz) ghee or coconut oil

1 cup (240 ml/8 fl oz) coconut milk or heavy whipping cream

4 cups (480 g/16.9 oz) uncooked Cauli-Rice (page 37)

NUTRITION FACTS PER SERVING

(4 meatballs + Cauli-Rice)

Total carbs: 11 g

Fiber: 4.2 g

Net carbs: 6.9 g

Protein: 30.6 g

Fat: 27.5 g

Energy: 410 kcal

Macronutrient ratio: Calories from carbs (7%), protein (31%), fat (62%)

Combine the minced chicken, coconut flour, egg, garlic, spices, and salt in a bowl. Using your hands, create medium-sized meatballs and set aside.

Heat the ghee in a large pan. When hot, drop in the meatballs. Cook for 3 minutes per side, turning until completely browned. Add the coconut milk and shake the pan to spread the milk. Cover with a lid and cook for about 10 minutes, until the meatballs are cooked through. (Cooking time depends on the size of the meatballs.)

Add the uncooked Cauli-Rice to the pan with the meatballs for the last 8 to 10 minutes of the cooking process or pan-fry and serve separately.

TIP

Make your own ground meat. Simply put the meat into a food processor and pulse until smooth. This allows you to choose the best cuts for your dishes and gives you complete control of what's on your plate. For best results with ground chicken, use chicken thighs—they're juicier and contain more fat than chicken breasts.

SIMPLE SHREDDED CHICKEN

This basic recipe yields two low-carb essentials that pop up in many of my recipes: tender chicken meat and homemade chicken stock.

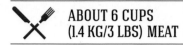 ABOUT 6 CUPS (1.4 KG/3 LBS) MEAT	5 MINS	3 TO 10 HOURS

INGREDIENTS

1 whole chicken (about 1.4 kg/ 3 lb, bone included)

2 quarts (2 L/67.6 fl oz) or more of water

Optional: ½ teaspoon salt or seasoning of your choice (e.g., bay leaf, paprika, curry powder, pepper)

NUTRITION FACTS PER SERVING

Total carbs: 0 g

Fiber: 0 g

Net carbs: 0 g

Protein: 27.9 g

Fat: 23.4 g

Energy: 322 kcal

Macronutrient ratio:
Calories from carbs (0%), protein (34.5%), fat (65.4%)

Wash the whole chicken in cold water and then pat it dry using a paper towel.

When boiling chicken in a regular pot: Place the chicken in the pot and fill with as much water as needed to cover the whole bird. Add your seasoning of choice and then cover the pot with a lid and bring the water to a boil. Next, reduce the heat to low and cook for at least an hour. The longer you cook the whole chicken, the more gelatin will be released from the joints and bones: I cook mine for about 3 hours. When done, the chicken should fall apart when scraped with a fork.

When using a slow cooker: Set the whole chicken into a slow cooker. For this method, you only need to use about ½ cup (120 ml/4.1 fl oz) water, but you can use more if you want to make more stock. Add your seasoning of choice and cook for 6 to 10 hours. Cooking time depends on your slow cooker: You can either cook it on high for about 6 hours, which I prefer, or low for up to 10 hours.

When the chicken is done, use tongs to transfer the whole chicken to a bowl to cool before shredding it. Use two forks or your hands to pull the meat off the bones and into bits. You can reuse the bones when making Bone Broth (page 30). Pour the chicken stock through a sieve and into airtight containers. Refrigerate for up to 3 days or freeze for up to 6 months.

CHICKEN CASSEROLE

All you need to make this filling chicken dish are a few basic low-carb ingredients.

6 SERVINGS	15 MINS	50 TO 55 MINS

INGREDIENTS

1.3 pounds (600 g) chicken thighs

¼ cup (56 g/2 oz) ghee or lard

1 small (70 g/2.5 oz) white onion

3 cups (300 g/10.6 oz) white mushrooms

1 medium (500 g/17.6 oz) head broccoli

2 large eggs

½ cup (120 ml/4 fl oz) heavy whipping cream

Pinch of salt

1 cup (150 g/5.3 oz) blue cheese, crumbled

½ cup (56 g/2 oz) cheddar cheese, shredded

Freshly ground black pepper

NUTRITION FACTS PER SERVING

Total carbs: 9.6 g

Fiber: 2.9 g

Net carbs: 6.7 g

Protein: 33.4 g

Fat: 32.2 g

Energy: 468 kcal

Macronutrient ratio:
Calories from carbs (6%), protein (29%), fat (65%)

Preheat the oven to 350°F (175°C, or gas mark 4). Dice the chicken thigh meat into medium-sized pieces. Grease a large pan with half the ghee, add the chicken, season with salt and black pepper, and cook over medium-high heat until browned on all sides. Place in a bowl and set aside.

Peel and slice the onion and wash and slice the mushrooms. Place the remaining ghee in the pan and, when hot, add the onion. Cook for about 3 minutes until translucent. Add the sliced mushrooms and cook for another 5 minutes, stirring frequently. Turn off the heat and set aside.

Wash the broccoli and cut it into small florets. (Don't throw away the broccoli stem; simply peel the hard skin off and chop the rest into small pieces.) Crack the eggs into a bowl and whisk with the cream and a pinch of salt.

Place all the ingredients in a large casserole dish: the broccoli florets, chopped broccoli stem, mushrooms, browned chicken, and eggs with cream. Add the crumbled blue cheese and combine well. Bake in the oven for 25 to 30 minutes.

Remove the casserole from the oven and top with the grated cheddar cheese. Return the dish to the oven, increase the temperature to 400°F (200°C, or gas mark 6) and cook for another 5 to 7 minutes. When done, remove the casserole from the oven and let it cool slightly before serving. Season with black pepper to taste.

TURKEY LEG WITH TARRAGON

Roasting turkey with butter crisps up the skin and makes the meat soft and juicy. It's a great source of potassium, too!

 4 SERVINGS | **10 MINS** | 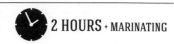 **2 HOURS** + MARINATING

INGREDIENTS

2 turkey legs, bone in
(1.8 kg/4 lb)

¼ cup (120 g/4.4 oz) ghee,
butter, or lard

1 bunch tarragon, about ¼ cup
(16 g/0.6 oz) chopped tarragon

1 tablespoon (6 g/0.2 oz)
fresh orange zest (or ½
tablespoon/3 g/0.1 oz dried)

Salt and freshly ground
black pepper

4 cloves garlic, crushed

½ cup (120 ml/4 fl oz) water,
or more if needed

NUTRITION FACTS
PER SERVING

Total carbs: 1.5 g

Fiber: 0.2 g

Net carbs: 1.2 g

Protein: 44.2 g

Fat: 28.9 g

Energy: 455 kcal

Macronutrient ratio:
Calories from carbs (1%),
protein (40%), fat (59%)

Pat the turkey dry with a kitchen towel and then rub in the ghee by lifting the turkey skin and massaging the ghee into the flesh. Rub more ghee on top of the skin and add chopped tarragon, orange zest, and crushed garlic. Season with salt and black pepper and let marinate in the fridge for at least 2 hours or overnight.

Remove the turkey from the fridge and keep at room temperature for about half an hour. Meanwhile, preheat the oven to 325°F (160°C, or gas mark 3). Set the turkey on a roasting rack in a roasting pan. Cover the pan with aluminum foil and place in the oven.

Cook for about 1 ½ hours, pouring the pan juices over the meat every half hour during the cooking process. Make sure the juices don't evaporate: pour in some water if needed. After 1 ½ hours of cooking, remove the foil and increase the temperature to 425°F (220°C, or gas mark 7). Continue to roast for another 30 minutes or until the meat thermometer reads 175°F (82°C).

When done, remove from the oven and let rest for 15 to 20 minutes before serving. Pour the cooking juices over the meat and pair with butter-roasted green beans or asparagus with a splash of lemon juice.

TIP

You can roast the whole bird with these ingredients, if you like—just double the amount of spices and herbs in this recipe. A 10-pound (4.6 kg) turkey will take 2½ to 3 hours to cook and will yield about 10 servings. If roasting a whole bird, let it rest for half an hour before serving: that's how it becomes really tender and succulent!

ROAST DUCK WITH BRAISED CABBAGE

Duck meat is tender, delicious, and keto-friendly if eaten with the skin on. And it's an amazing match for braised sweet-and-sour cabbage.

 4 SERVINGS   **20 MINS**   **2 HOURS**

INGREDIENTS

Duck

1 duck or 4 duck quarters (about 1.4 kg/3 lbs, bones included)

¼ teaspoon salt

Freshly ground black pepper

Braised Cabbage

½ head (300 g/10.6 oz) medium red cabbage, core removed

1 large (200 g/7.1 oz) turnip

1 small (70 g/2.5 oz) white onion

2 tablespoons (30 g/1.1 oz) ghee, lard, or duck fat

1½ cups (225 g/8 oz) sauerkraut, drained

¼ teaspoon ground cloves

2 tablespoons (30 ml/1 fl oz) apple cider vinegar

½ to 1 cup (240 ml/8 fl oz) chicken stock (page 128)

Salt and freshly ground black pepper, to taste

Preheat the oven to 400°F (200°C, or gas mark 6). Make sure you remove the giblets before cooking if using a whole duck.

Prick the duck's skin all over with the tip of a sharp knife and season with salt and black pepper. Place the duck on a rack in a roasting pan and roast the duck for 1 hour 20 minutes to 1 hour 30 minutes (or 20 minutes per every pound [455 g] plus 20 minutes extra). When done, cover with aluminum foil and leave to rest for 15 minutes.

While the duck is cooking, prepare the cabbage. Wash and slice the cabbage and peel and grate the turnip. Peel and finely slice the onion. Grease a large pot with ghee and add the onion. Cook until translucent and then add the shredded cabbage, turnip, and drained sauerkraut. Add the ground cloves, vinegar, and chicken stock and mix well. Season with salt and black pepper to taste. (If you're using a Dutch oven, you may not need any chicken stock, as only a small amount of water is lost during the cooking process.) Cover with a lid and cook on medium-low heat for about 30 minutes or until tender. Stir a few times to prevent burning.

When done, quarter the duck. Pour the duck fat in with the cabbage and mix well. Place the cabbage on a serving plate and top with the duck.

NUTRITION FACTS PER SERVING

Total carbs: 13 g   **Protein:** 25.9 g   **Macronutrient ratio:**
Fiber: 4.5 g   **Fat:** 46.5 g   Calories from carbs (6%), protein (19%), fat (75%)
Net carbs: 8.5 g   **Energy:** 568 kcal

TURKEY PATTIES WITH CUCUMBER SALSA

Throw these juicy turkey patties on the grill at your next summertime BBQ, then serve them alongside cucumber salsa and crispy greens.

16 PATTIES	15 MINS	20 MINS

INGREDIENTS

Turkey Patties

1.1 pounds (500 g) turkey, ground

½ cup (50 g/1.8 oz) almond flour

1 large egg

2 cloves garlic, crushed

1 small hot chile pepper, deseeded and

2 teaspoons Dijon Mustard (page 31)

2 tablespoons (30 ml/1 fl oz) lemon juice

2 tablespoons (8 g/0.3 oz) chopped fresh parsley

2 tablespoons (5 g/0.2 oz) chopped fresh basil

½ teaspoon salt

Freshly ground black pepper

2 medium (30 g/1.1 oz) spring onions, finely-sliced

2 tablespoons (30 g/1.1 oz) ghee or lard

(continued)

Put the turkey in a bowl and add the almond flour, egg, crushed garlic, chile pepper, Dijon mustard, lemon juice, parsley, basil, salt, and black pepper. Add one finely-sliced spring onion and leave the other for garnish. Mix all the ingredients until well combined and then use your hands to form small patties.

Heat the ghee in a griddle or regular pan and add the patties when hot. Don't turn the patties too soon or they will stick to the pan. Cook the patties on each side until browned, working in batches and placing on a plate one at a time as they get cooked. Set aside.

Meanwhile, prepare the cucumber salsa. Wash the cucumber and grate into a bowl. Wash and finely chop the jalapeño pepper. Add all the remaining ingredients, including the yogurt or sour cream, if using, and mix until well combined. Serve with the turkey patties.

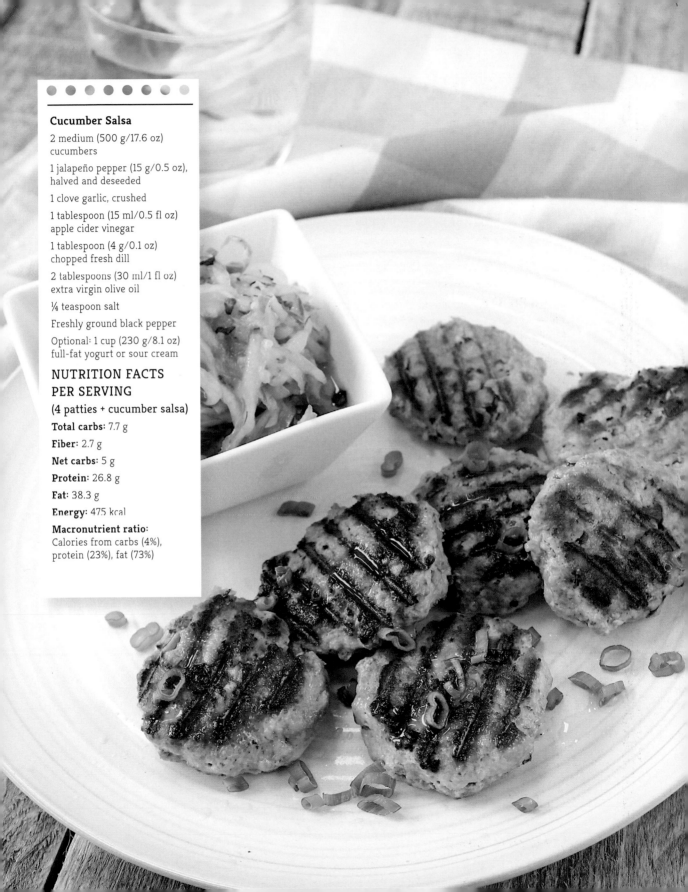

Cucumber Salsa

2 medium (500 g/17.6 oz) cucumbers

1 jalapeño pepper (15 g/0.5 oz), halved and deseeded

1 clove garlic, crushed

1 tablespoon (15 ml/0.5 fl oz) apple cider vinegar

1 tablespoon (4 g/0.1 oz) chopped fresh dill

2 tablespoons (30 ml/1 fl oz) extra virgin olive oil

¼ teaspoon salt

Freshly ground black pepper

Optional: 1 cup (230 g/8.1 oz) full-fat yogurt or sour cream

NUTRITION FACTS PER SERVING

(4 patties + cucumber salsa)

Total carbs: 7.7 g

Fiber: 2.7 g

Net carbs: 5 g

Protein: 26.8 g

Fat: 38.3 g

Energy: 475 kcal

Macronutrient ratio: Calories from carbs (4%), protein (23%), fat (73%)

BAKED SALMON & ASPARAGUS
WITH HOLLANDAISE

This simple, elegant, healthy low-carb meal is ready in less than half an hour!

 2 SERVINGS | **5 MINS** | **25 TO 30 MINS**

INGREDIENTS

2 large (400 g/14.1 oz) bunches asparagus

2 tablespoons (30 ml/1 fl oz) ghee or extra virgin olive oil

Salt and freshly ground black pepper, to taste

2 medium (300 g/10.6 oz) salmon fillets

2 servings Hollandaise Sauce (page 32)

NUTRITION FACTS PER SERVING

Total carbs: 9.5 g

Fiber: 4.3 g

Net carbs: 5.2 g

Protein: 39.9 g

Fat: 51.2 g

Energy: 649 kcal

Macronutrient ratio: Calories from carbs (3%), protein (25%), fat (72%)

Preheat the oven to 400°F (200°C, or gas mark 6). Clean the asparagus and snip off their woody ends. Arrange them on a baking sheet and toss with half of the ghee. Season with salt and pepper.

Place the salmon on another baking sheet and drizzle with the remaining ghee. Season with salt and black pepper and set in the oven, along with the asparagus, for 20 to 25 minutes.

While the fish and asparagus are baking, make the Hollandaise sauce. When done, place the asparagus and salmon on a serving plate and top with the Hollandaise sauce. Serve immediately.

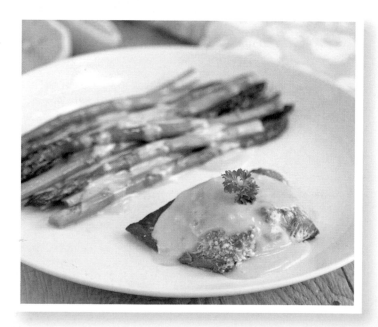

BAKED TUNA "PASTA"

Wide zucchini "noodles" offer a healthy alternative to pasta in this keto-friendly tuna bake.

 6 SERVINGS | **15 MINS** | **35 MINS**

INGREDIENTS

1 medium (100 g/3.5 oz) red onion

2 cups (200 g/7.1 oz) white mushrooms

¼ cup (56 g/2 oz) ghee or butter

3 medium (600 g/21.2 oz) zucchini

½ cup (125 g/4.4 oz) Pesto (page 35)

1 teaspoon dried oregano

2 teaspoons dried basil

3 cups (450 g/15.9 oz) canned tuna, drained

1 cup (110 g/3.9 oz) shredded mozzarella cheese

⅓ cup (30 g/1.1 oz) grated Parmesan cheese

Salt and freshly ground black pepper, to taste

NUTRITION FACTS PER SERVING

Total carbs: 8.1 g

Fiber: 2.4 g

Net carbs: 5.7 g

Protein: 29 g

Fat: 25.7 g

Energy: 375 kcal

Macronutrient ratio: Calories from carbs (6%), protein (31%), fat (63%)

Preheat the oven to 375°F (190°C, or gas mark 5). Peel and slice the onion and then wash and slice the mushrooms. Grease a pan with the ghee and add the onion. Cook until translucent and then add the sliced mushrooms. Cook for about 5 minutes more and remove from the heat.

Meanwhile, wash and thinly slice the zucchini using a potato peeler or a vegetable spiralizer to create wide flat noodles. Drop the noodles into a large casserole dish and add the mushrooms, pesto, herbs, seasonings, and tuna. Sprinkle with the mozzarella cheese and mix well.

Top with the grated Parmesan cheese and bake in the oven for about 20 minutes. When done, remove from the oven and let it cool slightly before serving.

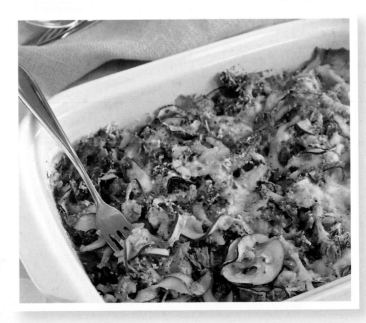

BRAISED SALMON
WITH SPINACH CREAM SAUCE

Salmon is a healthy fatty fish high in omega-3 fatty acids, and it's great with this silky spinach and cream sauce.

 4 SERVINGS | **15 MINS** | **35 MINS**

INGREDIENTS

Salmon

4 salmon filets (600 g/21.2 oz)

¼ teaspoon salt

2 tablespoon (30 ml/1 fl oz) lemon juice

Spinach cream sauce

3 tablespoons (45 g/1.5 oz) ghee or extra virgin olive oil

2 cloves garlic, crushed

2 medium (30 g/1.1 oz) spring onions, finely sliced

2 large bags spinach, fresh (400 g/14.1 oz) or frozen (435 g/15.3 oz)

½ cup (120 ml/2 fl oz) heavy whipping cream or coconut milk

1 cup (40 g/1.4 oz) fresh basil,

Salt and freshly ground black pepper, to taste

First, cook the salmon. Fill a steaming pot with about 2 inches (5 cm) of water. Bring the water to a boil over high heat. Season each salmon fillet with a pinch of salt and drizzle with fresh lemon juice. Reduce the heat to medium and place the salmon in the steaming basket. Cover with a lid and cook for 8 to 10 minutes or until the salmon flesh is opaque and separates easily with a fork.

Next, prepare the sauce. Wash and dry the spinach if using fresh. Heat the ghee in a pan and add the garlic and spring onion. Then, add the spinach and cook over medium heat for 1 to 2 minutes or until wilted. Pour in the cream and cook until it has reduced by about half. Add the finely chopped basil and a splash of lemon juice and season with salt and black pepper. Take it off the heat and set aside for 5 minutes.

To cream the sauce, use a hand blender or pour the mixture into a food processor and pulse until smooth. Set the salmon on a serving plate and top with the sauce. Serve with Shaved Asparagus with Parmesan Cheese (page 201) or Mediterranean Cauli-Rice (page 189).

NUTRITION FACTS PER SERVING

Total carbs: 5.9 g	**Protein:** 36.2 g	**Macronutrient ratio:** Calories from carbs (3%), protein (32%), fat (65%)
Fiber: 2.5 g	**Fat:** 32 g	
Net carbs: 3.5 g	**Energy:** 460 kcal	

SARDINE LETTUCE CUPS

Sardines are one of the most underestimated superfoods. They're high in healthy omega-3 fatty acids; they're sustainable and very reasonably priced; and their edible bones are rich in minerals!

4 SERVINGS	5 MINS	15 MINS

INGREDIENTS

12 to 15 fresh sardines or 6 tins of sardines (600 g/ 21.2 oz)

1 cup (150 g/5.3 oz) cherry tomatoes, chopped

1 large (150 g/5.3 oz) green pepper, sliced

1 medium (200 g/7.1 oz) cucumber, peeled and diced

1 small (60 g/2.1 oz) red onion

1 cup (150 g/5.3 oz) feta cheese

2 tablespoons (17 g/0.6 oz) capers

½ cup (50 g/1.8 oz) olives

1 tablespoon (15 ml/0.5 fl oz) lemon juice

1 teaspoon dried oregano

¼ cup (60 ml/2 fl oz) extra virgin olive oil

Salt and freshly ground black pepper, to taste

4 small (400 g/14.1 oz) heads lettuce

If using fresh sardines, preheat the oven to 350°F (175°C, or gas mark 4). Clean the sardines thoroughly, making sure to remove the gills and insides. Rinse under running water to wash off any scales and remaining blood. (You can also ask your local fishmonger to do the cleaning for you.) Set the sardines on a rack and season with salt and pepper. Bake for about 10 minutes. When done, remove from the oven and let them cool. Tear the meat off the bones and place in a bowl. If using canned sardines, drain the liquids out of the can and place the sardines in a bowl.

Peel and slice the red onion. In another bowl, mix the tomatoes, green bell pepper, cucumber, and red onion. Add the crumbled feta cheese, capers, olives, lemon juice, oregano, and olive oil. Season with salt and black pepper, if needed. Add the sardine meat and mix well.

Tear off the lettuce leaves and then wash and pat dry with a kitchen towel. Serve the sardines on top of the lettuce leaves or just fold everything into a bowl and serve.

NUTRITION FACTS PER SERVING

Total carbs: 10.3 g	**Protein:** 37.4 g	**Macronutrient ratio:** Calories from carbs (5%), protein (30%), fat (65%)
Fiber: 3.4 g	**Fat:** 36 g	
Net carbs: 6.9 g	**Energy:** 478 kcal	

DEVILED MACKEREL SKEWERS

Like sardines and salmon, mackerel is a keto-friendly superstar. It's high in omega-3 fatty acids, and it's so tasty that it rarely needs seasoning. Choose your fish carefully, though: some kinds of mackerel may have high mercury levels.

 4 SERVINGS   **10 MINS**   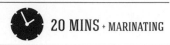 **20 MINS + MARINATING**

INGREDIENTS

6 mackerel fillets (600 g/21.2 oz)

2 cloves garlic, crushed

½ teaspoon flaked chile pepper or 1 teaspoon chopped fresh chile pepper

1 tablespoon (15 ml/0.5 fl oz) balsamic vinegar

¼ cup (60 ml/2 fl oz) extra virgin olive oil

1 medium (110 g/3.9 oz) white onion

2 large (300 g/10.6 oz) green peppers

2 medium (200 g/7.1 oz) red, orange, or yellow peppers

Salt and freshly ground black pepper, to taste

NUTRITION FACTS PER SERVING

Total carbs: 10.6 g

Fiber: 3 g

Net carbs: 7.6 g

Protein: 29.5 g

Fat: 34.8 g

Energy: 476 kcal

Macronutrient ratio: Calories from carbs (6%), protein (26%), fat (68%)

Slice the mackerel into medium pieces. Place in a bowl and add the crushed garlic, chili flakes, balsamic vinegar, and olive oil. Season with salt and black pepper and marinate for at least 1 hour or overnight.

Peel the onion and cut it into thick slices, thick enough to be able to pierce with a skewer. Wash, deseed, and slice the bell peppers into medium pieces.

Set the oven to broil (500°F [260°C, or gas mark 10]). Make the skewers by piercing the mackerel, onion, and bell peppers in an alternating order. Set the skewers on a rack in a roasting pan and transfer to the oven. Cook for 5 minutes and toss with some of the oil left over from marinating. Cook for another 5 minutes until browned. Serve immediately.

GRILLED TROUT WITH LEMON & HERB BUTTER

Try making your own herb butter: it's a snap, and it'll add healthy fats and extra flavor to lots of your meals.

 4 SERVINGS | **15 MINS** | **40 MINS**

INGREDIENTS

½ cup (110 g/3.9 oz) butter, room temperature

¼ cup (12 g/0.4 oz) chopped fresh herbs (e.g., basil, parsley, oregano, thyme)

4 cloves garlic, crushed

1 tablespoon (6 g/0.2 oz) freshly grated lemon zest

Salt and freshly ground black pepper, to taste

4 trout fillets (600 g/21.2 oz)

2 tablespoons (30 g/1.1 oz) ghee or coconut oil

NUTRITION FACTS PER SERVING

Total carbs: 1.9 g

Fiber: 0.5 g

Net carbs: 1.4 g

Protein: 31.3 g

Fat: 35 g

Energy: 452 kcal

Macronutrient ratio: Calories from carbs (1%), protein (28%), fat (71%)

First, prepare the herb butter by mixing the butter, freshly chopped herbs, crushed garlic cloves, lemon zest, salt, and black pepper. Make sure the butter is at room temperature; otherwise, it will be difficult to mix. Spoon the butter onto a piece of parchment paper and roll up to create a small parcel. Twist the sides of the paper and place in the fridge for at least 30 minutes.

Meanwhile, prepare the trout. Grease each fillet with some ghee and season with salt and black pepper. Heat a large griddle or regular pan over a medium-high heat and grease with the remaining ghee.

When the pan is hot, place the fish in the pan, skin-side down, and fry for 2 to 3 minutes or until the skin is crispy and browned. Avoid turning too soon, as the meat may stick to the pan. Turn on the other side and cook for another 2 minutes. Take the pan off of the heat and let the fish rest for 10 minutes. The residual heat will cook the trout through without overcooking it.

To serve, place the hot trout on a serving plate and add a few slices of the herb butter. Try it with Steamed Broccoli with Blue Cheese Sauce (page 95).

SWEET & SOUR CHILE PRAWNS

These zingy prawns can be a starter or a main course: just grab a grain-free tortilla, add the prawns plus your favorite low-carb fillings, and enjoy!

4 SERVINGS	15 MINS	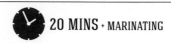 20 MINS + MARINATING

INGREDIENTS

¼ cup (56 g/2 oz) ghee or coconut oil

1 to 2 Thai chile peppers (45 g/1.6 oz)

4 cloves garlic, peeled and crushed

1 tablespoon (15 ml/0.5 fl oz) apple cider vinegar

2 tablespoons (30 g/1.1 oz) unsweetened tomato puree

2 tablespoons (30 ml/1 fl oz) fish sauce

1 bay leaf, crushed

1 teaspoon dried thyme

1 tablespoon (10 g/0.4 oz) erythritol or Swerve

5 to 10 drops liquid stevia

2 to 4 tablespoons (30 to 60 ml/1 to 2 fl oz) water

Salt and freshly ground black pepper, to taste

1.1 pounds (500 g) prawns, raw and peeled

1 bunch fresh cilantro and lime wedges, for garnish

Optional: Grain-free Tortillas (page 25)

First, make the chile sauce. Grease a large pan with the ghee. Wash, halve, and deseed the chile peppers and chop them into small pieces. Toss the chile peppers and garlic into the pan and cook for 2 to 3 minutes, stirring frequently. Add the apple cider vinegar, tomato puree, fish sauce, bay leaf, thyme, erythritol, liquid stevia, water, salt, and black pepper. Cook for another 5 minutes and keep stirring. Remove from the heat and let the sauce cool. Add the prawns (peeled, with or without tails) and coat in the chile sauce. Leave to marinate for at least an hour before cooking.

After marinating, return the pan to the heat and cook for just a few minutes until the prawns turn pink. (Alternatively, pierce the prawns with skewers and barbecue under a hot broiler.) Garnish with fresh cilantro and serve with lime wedges, leafy greens, sliced avocado, and Grain-Free Tortillas, if desired.

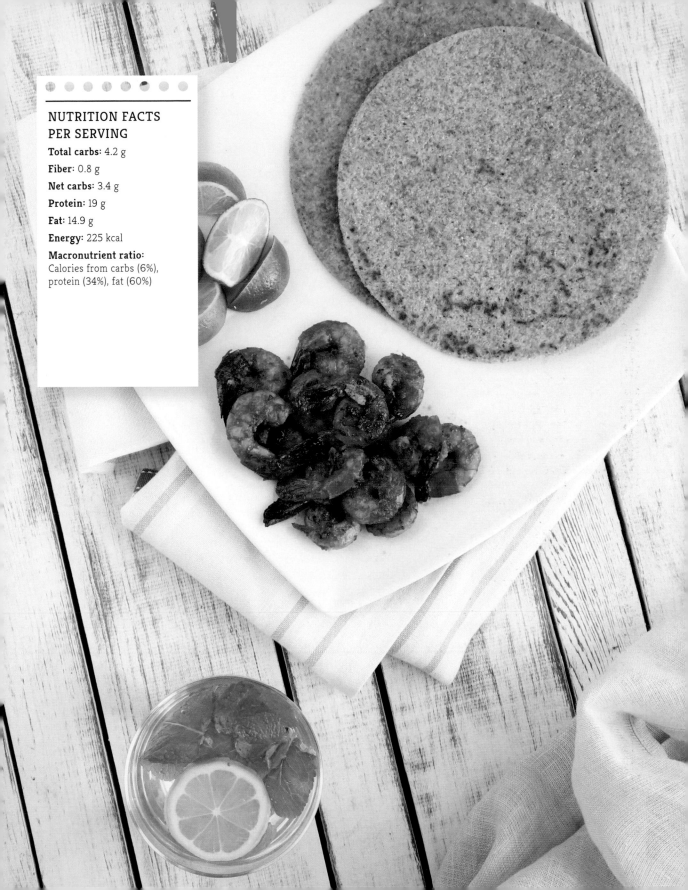

**NUTRITION FACTS
PER SERVING**

Total carbs: 4.2 g

Fiber: 0.8 g

Net carbs: 3.4 g

Protein: 19 g

Fat: 14.9 g

Energy: 225 kcal

Macronutrient ratio:
Calories from carbs (6%),
protein (34%), fat (60%)

HEALTHY FISH STICKS WITH TARTAR SAUCE

Beloved by kids everywhere, fish sticks are such a popular comfort food. Here, they get a healthy, low-carb makeover.

4 SERVINGS	15 MINS	45 MINS

INGREDIENTS

4 cod fillets, skinned and deboned (600 g/21.2 oz)

2 tablespoons (24 g/0.8 oz) coconut flour

1 large egg

1 tablespoon (15 ml/0.5 fl oz) freshly squeezed lemon juice

1 medium (15 g/0.5 oz) spring onion

3 tablespoons (20 g/0.7 oz) flax meal

⅓ cup (30 g/1.1 oz) grated Parmesan cheese, or pork rinds for a dairy-free alternative

½ teaspoon salt

Freshly ground black pepper, to taste

2 tablespoons (30 g/1.1 oz) ghee, melted, or coconut oil

(continued)

Preheat the oven to 400°F (200°C, or gas mark 6). Prepare the fish sticks. Place the cod in a blender and pulse until smooth. Transfer the blended cod to a bowl and add the coconut flour, egg, lemon juice, and the spring onion. Season with salt and black pepper and mix until well combined.

Prepare the breading by mixing the flax meal, Parmesan cheese, salt, and black pepper.

Using your hands, form 12 fish sticks (3 per serving). Roll each one in the breading until completely coated. Place on a baking sheet lined with parchment paper and drizzle with melted ghee. Transfer to the oven and bake for 25 to 30 minutes or until crispy and golden.

Meanwhile, prepare the slaw. Wash the cabbage and fennel. Using a sharp knife, finely slice the cabbage and fennel bulb or put both in a food processor and shred using a grating blade.

Set the shredded vegetables in a mixing bowl and add the spring onion. Finish with mayo and Dijon mustard and season with salt and black pepper. When done, set it aside.

Prepare the tartar sauce by mixing all the ingredients in a small bowl.

When the fish sticks are done, remove them from the oven and let them cool slightly. Serve with the slaw and tartar sauce.

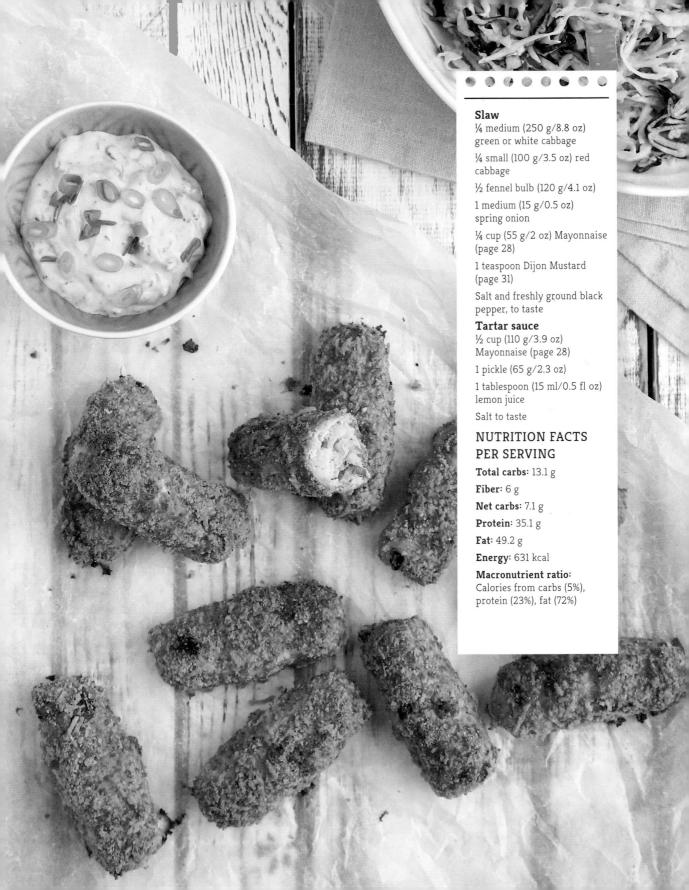

Slaw

¼ medium (250 g/8.8 oz) green or white cabbage

¼ small (100 g/3.5 oz) red cabbage

½ fennel bulb (120 g/4.1 oz)

1 medium (15 g/0.5 oz) spring onion

¼ cup (55 g/2 oz) Mayonnaise (page 28)

1 teaspoon Dijon Mustard (page 31)

Salt and freshly ground black pepper, to taste

Tartar sauce

½ cup (110 g/3.9 oz) Mayonnaise (page 28)

1 pickle (65 g/2.3 oz)

1 tablespoon (15 ml/0.5 fl oz) lemon juice

Salt to taste

NUTRITION FACTS PER SERVING

Total carbs: 13.1 g

Fiber: 6 g

Net carbs: 7.1 g

Protein: 35.1 g

Fat: 49.2 g

Energy: 631 kcal

Macronutrient ratio: Calories from carbs (5%), protein (23%), fat (72%)

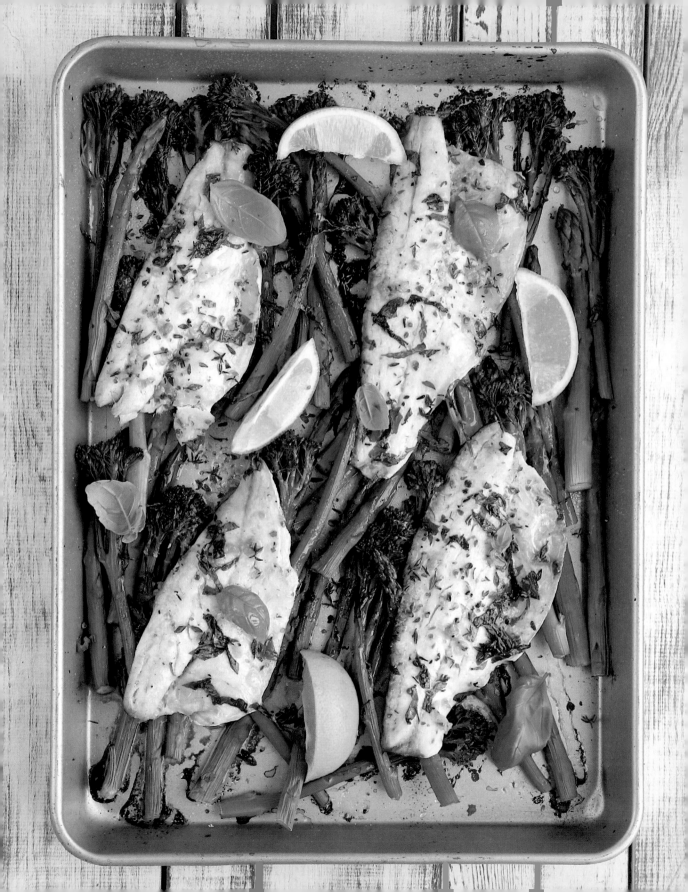

HERBED FISH & VEG TRAY

Light and delicious, this meal is also simple and doable: just about anyone can make it. Remember: when cooking with white fish like sea bass, always add some healthy fats like ghee or coconut oil to create a keto-friendly meal.

 4 SERVINGS | **5 MINS** | **20 MINS**

INGREDIENTS

3 cups (300 g/10.6 oz) broccoli

2 large bunches (300 g/10.6 oz) asparagus

4 large sea bass fillets (600 g/ 21.2 oz)

¼ cup (56 g/2 oz) ghee or butter

2 cloves garlic, crushed

Salt and freshly ground black pepper, to taste

¼ cup (12 g/0.4 oz) fresh herbs (basil, oregano, thyme) or 1 to 2 tablespoons dried herbs

1 teaspoon fresh lemon zest

2 tablespoons (30 ml/1 fl oz) freshly squeezed lemon juice

2 tablespoons (30 ml/1 fl oz) extra virgin olive oil

NUTRITION FACTS PER SERVING

Total carbs: 9.5 g

Fiber: 4 g

Net carbs: 5.6 g

Protein: 32.3 g

Fat: 26.4 g

Energy: 403 kcal

Macronutrient ratio: Calories from carbs (6%), protein (33%), fat (61%)

Preheat the oven to 350°F (175°C, or gas mark 4). Wash the broccoli and asparagus and place on a large baking sheet. Brush the sea bass with some of the ghee and rub in the crushed garlic.

Top the vegetables with the sea bass fillets and remaining melted ghee and season with salt and black black pepper. Sprinkle with chopped fresh herbs and lemon zest. Drizzle with the lemon juice and cook in the oven for about 15 minutes. When done, let the dish cool slightly and drizzle with extra virgin olive oil before serving.

SUSHI: SPICY TUNA ROLLS

Sushi lovers, rejoice: cauliflower rice can even be used to make sushi rolls!

4 SERVINGS	20 MINS	35 MINS

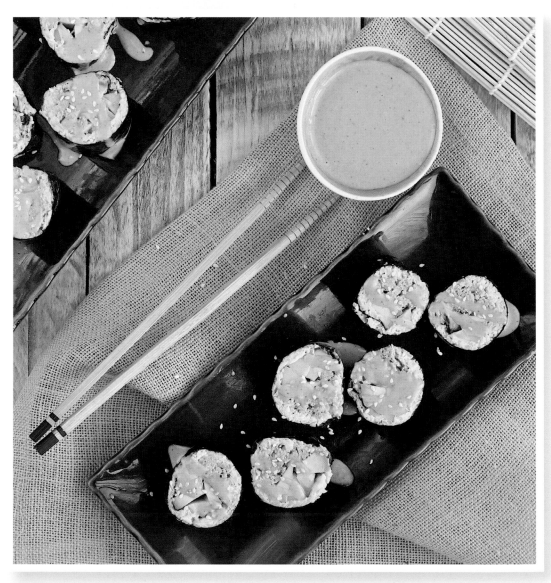

INGREDIENTS

½ small (56 g/2 oz) cucumber

1 large (200 g/7.1 oz) avocado

1 medium (15 g/0.5 oz) spring onion

1½ cups (220 g/8.1 oz) canned tuna, drained

2 cloves garlic, crushed

1 teaspoon grated ginger

2 teaspoons toasted sesame oil

¼ cup (55 g/1.9 oz) Mayonnaise (page 28)

4 cups (480 g/16.9 oz) Cauli-Rice (page 37)

2 teaspoons Sriracha

½ teaspoon salt

4 large (60 g/2.1 oz) leaves lettuce

4 nori seaweed sheets

Topping
¼ cup (55 g/1.9 oz) Mayonnaise (page 28)

1 teaspoon Sriracha

Salt and cayenne pepper to taste

2 tablespoons (16 g/0.6 oz) sesame seeds

NUTRITION FACTS PER SERVING
(1 uncut roll)

Total carbs: 15.6 g

Fiber: 8.4 g

Net carbs: 7.2 g

Protein: 21.5 g

Fat: 44.3 g

Energy: 523 kcal

Macronutrient ratio:
Calories from carbs (5%), protein (17%), fat (78%)

Wash, peel and slice the cucumber into long, thin stalks. Halve, deseed, and peel the avocado and cut into long slices. Wash the lettuce leaves and pat dry.

Wash and slice the spring onion. In another bowl, combine the drained tuna, sliced spring onion, crushed garlic, ginger, and sesame oil. Add 2 tablespoons (28 g/1 oz) of Mayonnaise, 2 teaspoons of Sriracha, and salt. Mix until well combined.

Add 2 tablespoons (28 g/1 oz) of Mayonnaise to the Cauli-Rice, and season with salt. Mix until well combined. The mayo will act as glue for the "rice."

Top each nori sheet with the cauli-rice. Make sure the cauli-rice doesn't cover the whole sheet; leave 1 to 2 inches (2.5 to 5 cm) on the sides. Top each sheet with a lettuce leaf, ¼ of the tuna mixture, ¼ of a sliced avocado, and ¼ of the cucumber. Make sure you place the filling on the top half of the nori so you can wrap it easily. Roll it up to the edge, wet the nori with a few drops of water, and seal well. Place the rolls with the sealed side down to keep the wraps tight. Leave to rest for 10 to 15 minutes before slicing or place in the fridge.

Meanwhile, prepare the topping. Mix the mayonnaise with the Sriracha and season with salt and cayenne pepper to taste. Dry-roast the sesame seeds for a minute or until golden. Cut each roll into 8 pieces and sprinkle with the toasted sesame seeds. Serve with the spicy mayonnaise.

ASIAN FISH BALLS WITH SWEET CHILI SAUCE

*White fish is naturally high in protein and low in fat. If
you need to increase your fat intake, make sure you include
a high-fat side like butter-roasted asparagus or broccoli.*

 16 FISH BALLS | **15 MINS** | **40 MINS**

INGREDIENTS

Fish Balls

4 fillets (600 g/21.2 oz) of
white fish such as cod, skinned
and deboned

1 large egg

½ cup (50 g/1.8 oz) almond flour

1 clove garlic, crushed

1 teaspoon freshly grated ginger

½ teaspoon salt

¼ cup (30 g/1.1 oz) coconut flour

Freshly ground black pepper

1 medium (15 g/0.5 oz)
spring onion

Optional: 2 tablespoons
(20 g/0.7 oz) toasted sesame
seeds, for garnish

Sweet Chili Sauce

¼ cup plus 2 tablespoons
(85 g/2 oz) ghee or coconut oil

1 small Thai chile pepper
(45 g/1.6 oz)

2 cloves garlic

1 teaspoon finely grated orange
zest (or ½ teaspoon dried)

¼ cup apple cider vinegar or
rice vinegar

2 tablespoons (26 g/0.9 oz)
fish sauce

1 tablespoon (15 ml/0.5 fl oz)
coconut aminos

1 tablespoon (15 ml/0.5 fl oz)
lime juice

(continued)

Preheat the oven to 400°F (200°C, or gas mark 6). Place the fish
in a blender and pulse until smooth. Transfer the fish to a bowl
and then add the egg, almond flour, crushed garlic, ginger, salt,
and black pepper.

Using your hands, form the mixture into small balls and roll
each fish ball in coconut flour until completely coated. Place on
a baking sheet lined with parchment paper. Transfer to the
oven and bake for 20 to 25 minutes.

Meanwhile, prepare the sweet chile sauce. Heat a large pan
greased with the ghee. Halve, deseed, and finely chop the chile
black pepper and peel and crush the garlic. Fry for 2 to 3
minutes and then add the orange zest, apple cider vinegar, fish
sauce, coconut aminos, lime juice, tomato puree, and erythritol
or liquid stevia. Season with salt and black pepper and cook over
medium heat for 5 to 10 minutes or until the sauce has reduced
by half. Then, remove from heat and add the ground chia seeds.
Mix until well combined and set aside to thicken.

When the fish balls are done, transfer them to the pan and
coat with the sauce. Serve immediately.

TIP

Serve with Cauli-Rice (page 37) or butter-roasted vegetables:
Try Asian-style vegetables such as steamed broccoli with dressing made
from freshly grated ginger, chile pepper, garlic, olive oil, toasted sesame
oil, and salt.

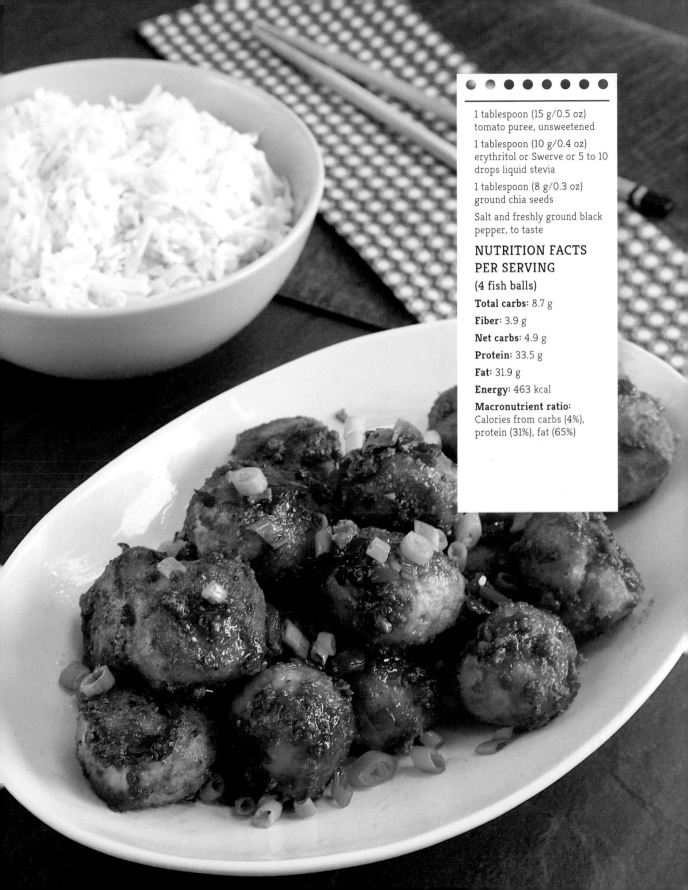

1 tablespoon (15 g/0.5 oz)
tomato puree, unsweetened

1 tablespoon (10 g/0.4 oz)
erythritol or Swerve or 5 to 10
drops liquid stevia

1 tablespoon (8 g/0.3 oz)
ground chia seeds

Salt and freshly ground black
pepper, to taste

NUTRITION FACTS PER SERVING

(4 fish balls)

Total carbs: 8.7 g

Fiber: 3.9 g

Net carbs: 4.9 g

Protein: 33.5 g

Fat: 31.9 g

Energy: 463 kcal

Macronutrient ratio:
Calories from carbs (4%),
protein (31%), fat (65%)

SLOW-COOKED BEEF KORMA

Make this popular Indian meal ahead and then eat it throughout the week with a side of Cauli-Rice (page 37).

 4 SERVINGS | **15 MINS** | **4 TO 6 HOURS**

INGREDIENTS

1.76 pounds (800 g) beef—any cut suitable for slow-cooking, such as braising steak, brisket, or chuck

½ medium (55 g/1.9 oz) white onion

1 clove garlic

1 tablespoon (8 g/0.05 oz) ginger

1 tablespoon (15 g/0.5 oz) tallow, lard, or ghee

2 whole cardamom pods

1 teaspoon ground turmeric

½ teaspoon ground coriander seeds

1 teaspoon garam masala spice mix

½ teaspoon salt, or more to taste

Freshly ground black pepper

½ cup (120 ml/4 fl oz) coconut milk or heavy whipping cream

¼ cup (60 ml/2 fl oz) water

Optional: 4 cups (480 g/16.9 oz) Cauli-Rice (page 37)

Dice the meat into medium-sized pieces. Peel and dice the onion, mash the garlic, and grate the ginger.

Grease a heavy-bottomed pan with tallow (or ghee or lard, but you can use tallow from the Bone Broth recipe on page 30—it's one of the great by-products of making Bone Broth). Add the chopped onion, garlic, and ginger. Cook for about 3 minutes on medium-high heat, stirring frequently.

Increase the temperature and add the meat. Cook until slightly browned on all sides. Spoon everything from the pan into a slow cooker and add all the spices, salt, and black pepper.

Pour in the coconut milk and water and stir well. (If you're using cream, add it at the end of the cooking process; otherwise, it will break down.) Cook for 4 to 6 hours on high or up to 10 hours on low. The exact time depends on the slow cooker. If you don't have a slow cooker, use a regular deep, heavy-bottomed casserole dish and cook in an oven preheated to 300°F (150°C, or gas mark 2) for 4 to 6 hours. When done, the meat should be soft and falling apart.

TIP

Make your own Garam Masala at home! Simply mix 1 tablespoon (7 g/0.3 oz) of ground cumin, 1½ teaspoons ground coriander seeds, 1½ teaspoons ground cardamom seeds, ½ teaspoon ground cloves, ½ teaspoon nutmeg, 1 teaspoon cinnamon, and 1½ teaspoons freshly ground black pepper.

NUTRITION FACTS PER SERVING

Total carbs: 3.6 g | **Protein:** 36.8 g | **Macronutrient ratio:** Calories from carbs (2%), protein (23%), fat (75%)
Fiber: 0.7 g | **Fat:** 54.1 g |
Net carbs: 2.9 g | **Energy:** 654 kcal |

CUBAN SHREDDED BEEF (ROPA VIEJA)

This popular Cuban meal is so flexible: it goes well with Cauli-Rice, and you can also add it to salads or use it as a filling for Essential Keto Crepes.

 4 SERVINGS | **15 MINS** | **4 TO 6 HOURS**

INGREDIENTS

2 cloves garlic, peeled and diced

1 small (70 g/2.5 oz) white onion, peeled and diced

1 jalapeño pepper (15 g/0.5 oz)

1 tablespoon (15 g/0.5 oz) ghee, lard, or tallow

1.76 pounds (800 g) beef, braising steak, or brisket

2 medium (240 g/8.5 oz) green peppers, sliced

1 bay leaf

1 teaspoon dried oregano

1 teaspoon dried thyme

½ teaspoon salt, or more to taste

2 tablespoons (30 ml/1 fl oz) lime juice

½ cup (120 ml/4 fl oz) Bone Broth (page 30) or vegetable stock

½ cup (120 ml/4 fl oz) tomato sauce (passata), unsweetened

Fresh cilantro, for garnish

Optional: 4 cups (480 g/16.9 oz) Cauli-Rice (page 37)

Wash, halve, deseed, and dice the jalapeno pepper. Place the garlic, onion, and jalapeño in a pan greased with ghee (or coconut oil) and cook for about 3 minutes, stirring frequently, until slightly golden. When done, set it aside.

Place the meat in the slow cooker and add the green bell pepper and all the spices. Squeeze in the lime juice and add the Bone Broth or vegetable stock. Add the fried onion, garlic, and jalapeño pepper and season with salt. Pour the passata over the roast.

Cook for 4 to 6 hours on high or up to 10 hours on low. The exact time depends on the slow cooker, so check the meat while it cooks. Pull the meat apart by tearing it into thin shreds with two forks. Garnish with the cilantro.

Serve with plain Cauli-Rice or green beans: you can either cook them separately, or add them to the meat for the last 2 to 3 hours in the slow cooker. To store, let it cool, transfer the meat into an airtight container, and keep it in the fridge for up to 5 days.

TIP

If you don't have a slow cooker, use a regular deep, heavy-bottom casserole dish and cook in the oven preheated to 300°F (150°C, or gas mark 2) for 4 to 6 hours.

NUTRITION FACTS PER SERVING

Total carbs: 8.1 g   **Protein:** 37.7 g

Fiber: 2.4 g   **Fat:** 48.8g

Net carbs: 5.7 g   **Energy:** 627 kcal

Macronutrient ratio: Calories from carbs (4%), protein (25%), fat (71%)

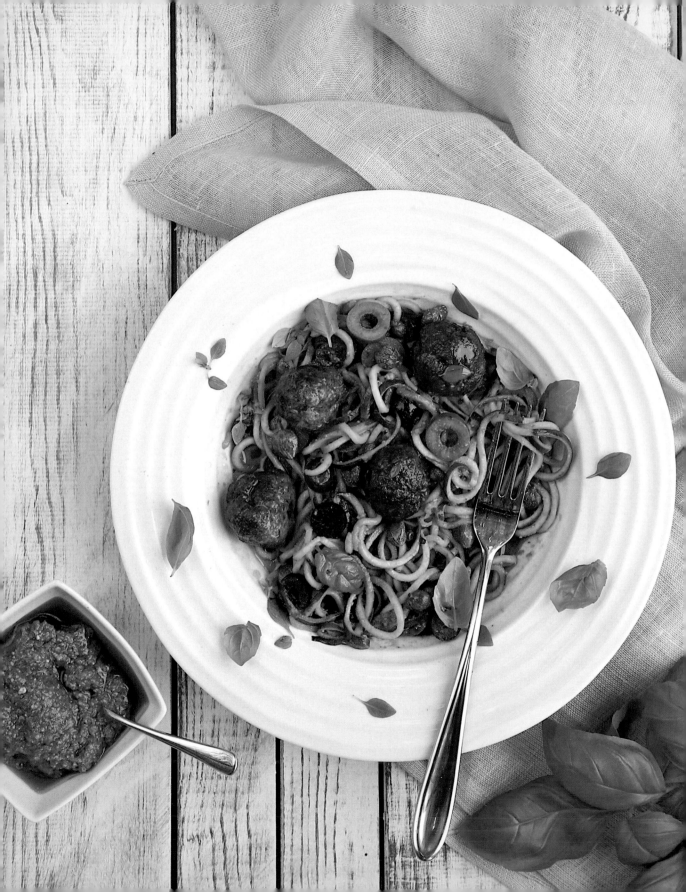

BEEF MEATBALLS WITH "ZOODLES"

Pesto, capers, and olives pep up this healthy take on spaghetti and meatballs.

 16 MEATBALLS | **15 MINS** | **20 MINS**

INGREDIENTS

1.1 pounds (500 g) ground beef

1 large egg

½ cup (50 g/1.8 oz) almond flour

½ cup (125 g/4.4 oz) Pesto (page 35)

2 tablespoons (5 g/0.2 oz) chopped fresh basil, plus more for garnish

1 tablespoon (15 g/0.5 oz) ghee or lard

4 medium (800 g/1.76 lb) zucchini

4 tablespoons (35 g/1.2 oz) capers

½ cup (50 g/1.8 oz) kalamata or green olives, pitted and sliced

½ teaspoon salt, or more to taste

Optional: ½ cup (45 g/1.6 oz) grated Parmesan cheese

NUTRITION FACTS PER SERVING
(4 meatballs + zoodles)

Total carbs: 11.9 g

Fiber: 5 g

Net carbs: 6.8 g

Protein: 29.8 g

Fat: 56.1 g

Energy: 659 kcal

Macronutrient ratio: Calories from carbs (4%), protein (18%), fat (78%)

Place the ground beef, egg, and almond flour into a mixing bowl. Add half of the pesto sauce and the basil. Season with salt and black pepper and process well. Using your hands, create small meatballs and set aside.

Heat a large pan greased with ghee. Once hot, add the meatballs. Cook for 2 to 3 minutes on one side over a medium-high heat and then turn using a fork. Keep turning until the meatballs are browned on all sides. When done, transfer the meatballs to a bowl and keep warm.

Wash the zucchini and use a julienne peeler or a vegetable spiralizer to create thin zucchini "noodles." Set them in the pan you used for making the meatballs and cook over a medium-high heat for 3 to 5 minutes. Remove from the heat and add the remaining pesto sauce, capers, and sliced olives. Mix until well combined and season with salt, if needed.

To serve, place the zoodles on a serving plate and top with the cooked meatballs. Garnish with the remaining basil leaves. Sprinkle with the Parmesan cheese, if using.

ASIAN SPICED BEEF MEATBALLS

It's impossible to eat just one of these herbed Asian meatballs. Serve them with my sweet-and-spicy chile sauce, plus a side of freshly-cut vegetables.

 16 MEATBALLS | **15 MINS** | **20 MINS**

INGREDIENTS

Meatballs

2 medium (30 g/1.1 oz) spring onions

1.1 pounds (500 g) ground beef

2 cloves garlic, crushed

2 tablespoons (30 ml/1 fl oz) fish sauce

1 teaspoon finely chopped lemongrass or organic lime zest

2 tablespoons (12 g/0.4 oz) chopped fresh mint

2 tablespoons (30 g/1.1 oz) ghee or coconut oil

Salt and freshly ground black pepper, to taste

2 tablespoons (18 g/0.6 oz) toasted sesame seeds

Spicy Dip

1 medium (15 g/0.5 oz) spring onion

1 clove garlic, crushed

1 teaspoon ginger

1 small hot chile pepper

1 tablespoon (1 g/0.04 oz) chopped fresh cilantro

1 tablespoon (15 ml/0.5 fl oz) fresh lime juice

2 tablespoons (30 ml/1 fl oz) coconut aminos

1 teaspoon toasted sesame oil

1 tablespoon (10 g/0.4 oz) erythritol or Swerve or 3 to 5 drops stevia

Salt and freshly ground black pepper, to taste

Wash and finely chop the spring onions. Place all the ingredients for the meatballs except the ghee in a mixing bowl and combine well. Using your hands, form small meatballs and set aside.

Heat a large pan greased with ghee. Add the meatballs and cook over a medium-high heat for 2 to 3 minutes and then turn using a fork. Keep turning until the meatballs are completely browned. When done, transfer the meatballs to a bowl and keep warm.

Meanwhile, prepare the dip. Wash and slice the spring onion. Mix all the ingredients for the dip and season with salt and black pepper to taste. Instead of erythritol or stevia, you can use 1 teaspoon of yacon syrup (page 17). Serve the meatballs with the dip immediately.

TIP

These meatballs are delicious with freshly-chopped vegetables such as cucumber and bell peppers.

NUTRITION FACTS PER SERVING (4 meatballs)

Total carbs: 4.4 g | **Protein:** 23.2 g | **Macronutrient ratio:** Calories from carbs (3%), protein (22%), fat (75%)
Fiber: 1.1 g | **Fat:** 35.9 g |
Net carbs: 3.3 g | **Energy:** 437 kcal |

BEEF TERIYAKI LETTUCE CUPS

Tender, juicy steak with sugar-free teriyaki sauce makes for a low-carb variation of a popular Asian dish. And it looks great as a party snack, too.

 4 SERVINGS | **15 MINS** | **20 MINS**

INGREDIENTS

2 small (200 g/7.1 oz) red, orange, or yellow peppers

1 medium (150 g/5.3 oz) green pepper

1 cup (100 g/3.5 oz) white mushrooms

1 small (70 g/2.5 oz) white onion

2 cloves garlic, crushed

2 teaspoons grated ginger

1 small hot chile pepper

2 large (600 g/21.2 oz) steaks (sirloin, rump, or flank)

¼ cup (56 g/2 oz) ghee or coconut oil

¼ cup (60 ml/2 fl oz) coconut aminos

3 tablespoons (45 ml/14.4 fl oz) fish sauce

1 tablespoon (8 g/0.3 oz) ground chia seeds

2 tablespoons (30 ml/1 fl oz) lime juice

1 teaspoon toasted sesame oil

Salt and freshly ground black pepper, to taste

2 medium (300 g/10.6 oz) heads green lettuce

First, prepare the vegetables. Wash, halve, and deseed the bell peppers and cut them into medium slices. Wash and slice the mushrooms and peel and slice the onion. Peel and crush the garlic and grate the ginger. Wash, halve, deseed, and finely chop the chile pepper. Wash the lettuce leaves and pat dry.

Cut the beef into thin slices. Heat a large pan over a medium-high heat and grease with the ghee. Once hot, add the beef and season with salt and black pepper. Keep stirring until the beef is browned from all sides, about 2 to 3 minutes. Transfer the beef into a bowl and keep warm.

Return the pan to the heat and add the garlic, ginger, and chile pepper. Cook for about 1 to 2 minutes, stirring frequently. Add the coconut aminos and fish sauce. Add the erythritol and stevia, if using. Add the ground chia seeds, stirring frequently. Keep cooking until the sauce thickens and has reduced by half.

Add the sliced bell peppers, mushrooms, onion, and lime juice. Mix well to coat with sauce. Cook for an additional 5 minutes or until the vegetables are tender yet still crisp.

Add the cooked beef and remove the pan from the heat. Drizzle with toasted sesame oil and set aside. Serve over separated lettuce leaves such as Romaine or Little Gem. Alternatively, use this recipe as a filling in Grain-Free Tortillas (page 25) or eat it with Cauli-Rice (page 28).

NUTRITION FACTS PER SERVING

Total carbs: 13.1 g   **Protein:** 35 g

Fiber: 4.6 g   **Fat:** 32.7 g

Net carbs: 8.5 g   **Energy:** 490 kcal

Macronutrient ratio: Calories from carbs (7%), protein (30%), fat (63%)

ULTIMATE GUACBURGER

This delicious keto burger is loaded with healthy fats and electrolytes which will help you overcome "keto-flu" during the first few days of the ketogenic diet (page 11).

 4 BURGERS | 15 MINS | 25 MINS

INGREDIENTS

Serve with 4 Ultimate Keto Buns (page 26); prepare ahead and save the rest of the buns for another meal

Burger Meat

1.1 pounds (500 g) ground beef

1 teaspoon Dijon Mustard (page 31)

1 tablespoon (15 g/0.5 oz) Ketchup (page 29) or Spicy Chocolate BBQ Sauce (page 34)

½ teaspoon garlic powder

½ teaspoon onion powder

½ teaspoon salt, or more to taste

Freshly ground black pepper

2 tablespoons (30 g/1.1 oz) ghee, tallow, or lard

(continued)

Make the Ultimate Keto Buns.

For the burgers, mix the ground beef with the mustard, ketchup, garlic powder, onion powder, salt, and black pepper. Create four small, palm-sized burgers.

Preheat a large pan greased with ghee. When hot, add the burgers. Turn the heat down to medium and cook on each side for 4 to 5 minutes: don't turn the meat too soon or it will stick to the pan. Use a spatula to lightly press the burgers down while cooking. When done, set them aside.

Meanwhile, prepare the guacamole. Halve and peel the avocado, remove the seed, and scoop half of the avocado meat into a bowl. Mash it well using a fork. Add the onion and lime juice, followed by the tomatoes, cilantro, crushed garlic, and chile pepper.

Dice the rest of the avocado and mix into the salad—do not mash! Season the salad with salt and black pepper to taste.

Cut each of the Ultimate Keto Buns in half and brown in a griddle pan for 2 to 3 minutes. Top with the burger and the prepared guacamole salad. If you're not serving the guacamole immediately, make sure you keep it in an airtight container to keep the avocado from browning.

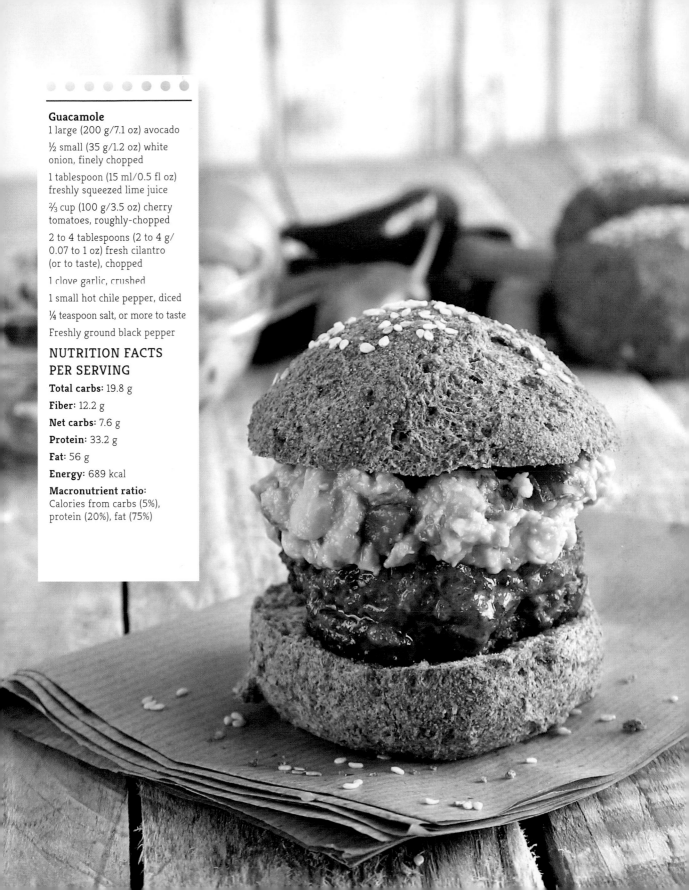

Guacamole

1 large (200 g/7.1 oz) avocado

½ small (35 g/1.2 oz) white onion, finely chopped

1 tablespoon (15 ml/0.5 fl oz) freshly squeezed lime juice

⅔ cup (100 g/3.5 oz) cherry tomatoes, roughly-chopped

2 to 4 tablespoons (2 to 4 g/ 0.07 to 1 oz) fresh cilantro (or to taste), chopped

1 clove garlic, crushed

1 small hot chile pepper, diced

¼ teaspoon salt, or more to taste

Freshly ground black pepper

NUTRITION FACTS PER SERVING

Total carbs: 19.8 g

Fiber: 12.2 g

Net carbs: 7.6 g

Protein: 33.2 g

Fat: 56 g

Energy: 689 kcal

Macronutrient ratio: Calories from carbs (5%), protein (20%), fat (75%)

SUCCULENT STEAK WITH CHIMICHURRI SAUCE

Everyone should know how to make a perfect steak. This one is so easy, and it's delicious with vibrant Argentinian chimichurri!

2 SERVINGS	20 MINS	25 MINS

INGREDIENTS

Steak

2 medium (400 g/14.1 oz) rib-eye steaks

2 teaspoons ghee, lard, or tallow

¼ teaspoon salt

Freshly ground black pepper

Chimichurri

2 cloves garlic

½ cup (15 g/0.5 oz) chopped fresh parsley

2 tablespoons (8 g/0.3 oz) chopped fresh oregano

1 small hot chile pepper

1 tablespoon (15 ml/0.5 fl oz) red or white wine vinegar

¼ cup (60 ml/2 fl oz) extra virgin olive oil

¼ teaspoon salt or more to taste

Freshly ground black pepper

(continued)

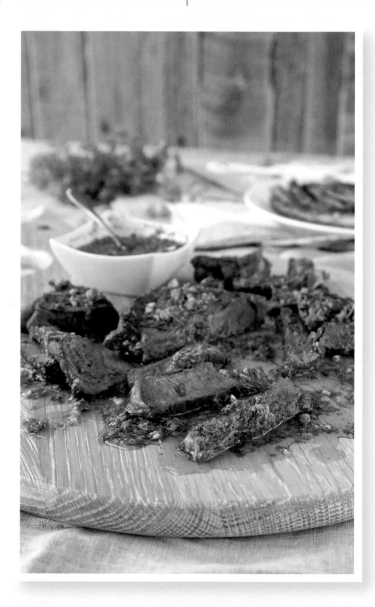

Buttered asparagus

2 medium (250 g/8.8 oz) bunches asparagus

1 tablespoon (15 g/0.5 oz) ghee or butter

¼ teaspoon salt

Freshly ground black pepper

2 tablespoons (30 ml/1 fl oz) lemon juice

NUTRITION FACTS PER SERVING

Total carbs: 10 g

Fiber: 4.3 g

Net carbs: 5.7 g

Protein: 41.1 g

Fat: 76.3 g

Energy: 883 kcal

Macronutrient ratio:
Calories from carbs (2%), protein (19%), fat (79%)

Allow the steak to sit at room temperature for 10 to 15 minutes while you prepare the chimichurri sauce. Peel the garlic and roughly chop the parsley and oregano. Wash, halve, and deseed the chile pepper. Place half of the parsley, oregano, and oil into a blender; set the rest aside for later. Add the vinegar, salt, and black pepper. Pulse a few times until smooth and then add the remaining herbs and oil. Mix until well combined. Meanwhile, set the oven to broil (500°F [260°C, or gas mark 10]).

Using a paper towel, pat the excess blood from the steaks. Toss with some of the melted ghee (or butter, tallow, or lard) and season with salt and black pepper. Make sure you season the steak after you toss it with the melted ghee: You don't want to wash the seasoning off.

Fry the steaks in a very hot heavy-based pan greased with ghee over high heat for 2 to 4 minutes on each side to seal in the juices. When you see the sides browning, it's time to flip it over. The exact time depends on the size of your steak; for example, a small one would take 2 minutes, while a large one could take up to 4 minutes to brown.

Reduce the heat to medium and continue to cook for another 4 minutes (rare), 7 minutes (medium), or 11 minutes (well done). There is no need to turn the steak again.

Remove the steak from the pan and allow it to rest in a warm place for 5 to 7 minutes. The steak will finish cooking in its residual heat as the temperature slowly lowers. The best way to rest the steak is to fold it up in parchment paper and then in a kitchen towel. This will keep it juicy and equally pink inside.

While the steak is resting, prepare the buttered asparagus. Snip the woody ends off of the vegetables. Set the asparagus into a bowl and toss with the ghee, salt, and black pepper. Place it on a rack or in a baking sheet and broil for 5 to 7 minutes. When ready, the asparagus should be tender and slightly browned yet still crisp. Remove from the oven and add a squeeze of lemon juice.

Place the rested steak on a plate, top with chimichurri sauce, and serve with the buttered asparagus.

ITALIAN "MEATZA"

*"Meatza" is pizza with a crust made from ground meat.
It's very low in carbs, and it's best with vegetable and cheese toppings.*

4 SERVINGS	15 MINS	25 TO 30 MINS

INGREDIENTS

Pizza Crust

1.1 pounds (500 g) ground beef

1 teaspoon each dried oregano and basil

½ teaspoon salt

Freshly ground black pepper

Toppings

2 cups (200 g/7.1 oz) wild mushrooms or ½ cup (50 g/ 1.8 oz) dried porcini mushrooms, soaked

2 tablespoons (30 g/1.1 oz) ghee

2 cloves garlic, crushed

1 large package spinach, fresh (200 g/7.1 oz) or frozen and defrosted (220 g/7.7 oz)

Salt and freshly ground black pepper, to taste

2 tablespoons (30 g/1.1 oz) Pesto (page 35)

¾ cup (100 g/3.5 oz) shredded mozzarella cheese

Preheat the oven to 400°F (200°C, or gas mark 6). In a bowl, combine the ground beef, oregano, basil, salt, and black pepper and mix well. You can either make one large pizza or 4 individual/ mini pizzas (which are easy to freeze for later). Using your hands, form the pizza "crust," making it about half an inch (1 cm) thick. Place on a baking sheet lined with parchment paper. Place in the oven and cook for 10 minutes.

Meanwhile, prepare the toppings. Wash and slice the mushrooms. If you are using dried mushrooms, soak them for at least 15 minutes before adding to the pan. Wash and dry the spinach if using fresh. Heat a large pan greased with the ghee and add the crushed garlic. Cook for one minute.

Add the mushrooms and cook for 5 minutes, stirring frequently. Toss in the fresh spinach and cook for one more minute. Season with salt and black pepper to taste. If you're using frozen spinach, make sure it's defrosted and squeeze any excess water out before cooking. Remove the pan from the heat.

When the meat crust is cooked, remove it from the oven and spread the pesto sauce on top. Add half of the mozzarella cheese and all of the spinach and mushroom mixture. Finish with the remaining mozzarella cheese and return to the oven for 5 minutes or until the cheese is melted.

NUTRITION FACTS PER SERVING

Total carbs: 5.6 g   **Protein:** 30.8 g   **Macronutrient ratio:** Calories from carbs (3%), protein (24%), fat (73%)

Fiber: 2.3 g   **Fat:** 41.7 g

Net carbs: 3.4 g   **Energy:** 520 kcal

OXTAIL CASSEROLE

Oxtail is one of the most underestimated cuts of beef. If cooked properly in a slow cooker, it's delicious, juicy, and high in gelatin—perfect for making Bone Broth!

 6 SERVINGS | **10 MINS** | **2 HOUR 45 MIN** + MARINATING

INGREDIENTS

¼ cup (56 g/2 oz) ghee

2 cloves garlic, crushed

1 small (70 g/2.5 oz) white onion, finely sliced

3 pounds (1.4 kg) oxtail, bone in

1 teaspoon cinnamon

¼ teaspoon ground cloves

2 bay leaves

2 tablespoons (5 g/0.2 oz) fresh thyme leaves

1 teaspoon salt or to taste

Freshly ground black pepper

1 small can (200 g/7.1 oz) diced tomatoes

2 cups (480 ml/16 fl oz) Bone Broth (page 30)

1 cup (240 ml/8.1 fl oz) water

3 cups (300 g/10.6 oz) green beans

2 large (400 g/14.1 oz) turnips

NUTRITION FACTS PER SERVING

Total carbs: 11.4 g

Fiber: 3.5 g

Net carbs: 7.9 g

Protein: 39.3 g

Fat: 36.8 g

Energy: 539 kcal

Macronutrient ratio: Calories from carbs (6%), protein (30%), fat (64%)

You can make the casserole in a Dutch oven, an ovenproof heavy soup pot, or in a slow cooker.

If using a Dutch oven or a heavy soup pot: Grease the Dutch oven with ghee and add the crushed garlic and finely-sliced onion. Cook for a few minutes until translucent. Add the oxtail and brown on all sides. Add the cinnamon, cloves, bay leaves, and thyme and season with salt and black pepper. Add the canned tomatoes and pour in the Bone Broth and water. Bring to a boil and reduce the heat to minimum. Cover with a lid and cook for 3 to 3½ hours or until the meat is tender. Check every hour in case more water is needed.

Meanwhile, prepare the vegetables. Trim the green beans and chop them into quarters. Peel and slice the turnip and dice into medium pieces.

When the oxtail is tender, use a slotted spoon to transfer it to a plate and let it rest until cool enough to handle. Shred the meat using your hands and a fork. Set the shredded meat aside. Reserve the bones for making more Bone Broth.

Add the chopped green beans and diced turnips to the pot with the oxtail juices and bring to a boil. Reduce the heat, cover with a lid, and cook for 45 to 60 minutes or until tender. When done, add the shredded meat.

If using a slow cooker: In a large pot, brown the garlic, onion, and oxtail and then transfer to the slow cooker. Add the spices, salt, black pepper, tomatoes, Bone Broth, and water and cook for 6 hours on high or 10 hours on low. Add the green beans and turnips for the last 2 to 3 hours of cooking.

PERFECT RIB EYE WITH HORSERADISH SAUCE

What could be better than perfectly-cooked, juicy steak marinated in garlic and served with sharp horseradish sauce?

 2 SERVINGS | **20 MINS** | **25 MINS**

INGREDIENTS

Steak

2 medium (400 g/14.1 oz) grass-fed rib-eye steaks

2 teaspoons ghee, lard, or tallow

2 cloves garlic, crushed

¼ teaspoon salt

Pinch cayenne pepper

Horseradish Sauce

2 tablespoons (30 g/1.1 oz) Mayonnaise (page 28)

2 tablespoons (30 g/1.1 oz) sour cream or more Mayonnaise

2 tablespoons (15 ml/0.5 fl oz) heavy whipping cream or coconut milk

1 to 2 tablespoons (15 to 30 g/ 0.5 to 1.1 oz) freshly grated horseradish

1 tablespoon (15 ml/0.5 fl oz) lemon juice

1 medium (15 g/0.5 oz) spring onion or chives

Salt and freshly ground black pepper, to taste

Allow the steak to sit at room temperature for 10 to 15 minutes. Using a paper towel, pat off the excess blood. Toss with some of the melted ghee and crushed garlic and season with salt and cayenne pepper. Let it marinate in the fridge for at least an hour.

Over high heat, fry the steak in a very hot heavy-based pan greased with ghee for 2 to 4 minutes on each side to seal in the juices. When you see the sides getting brown, it's time to flip it over. The exact time depends on the size of your steak. Small would take about 2 minutes to brown, while a large could take up to 4 minutes.

Reduce the heat to medium and continue to cook for another 4 minutes (rare), 7 minutes (medium), or 11 minutes (well done). There is no need to turn the steak again.

Remove the steak from the pan and allow it to rest in a warm place for 5 to 7 minutes. The steak will finish cooking from its residual heat as the temperature slowly goes down. The best way to rest the steak is to fold it up in parchment paper and then wrap it in a kitchen towel. This will keep it juicy and equally pink inside.

While the steak is resting, prepare the horseradish sauce: Combine all the ingredients in a bowl and mix well. Place the rested steak on a plate and serve with the horseradish sauce and vegetable sides.

NUTRITION FACTS PER SERVING

Total carbs: 4.4 g **Protein:** 38.7 g **Macronutrient ratio:** Calories from carbs (2%), protein (22%), fat (76%)
Fiber: 0.8 g **Fat:** 61 g
Net carbs: 3.6 g **Energy:** 721 kcal

PERFECTLY PULLED PORK

Making slow-cooked meat in advance is a smart way to save time. Make this recipe on a weekend and use it throughout the week on omelets, in low-carb tortillas and enchiladas, or on its own with vegetable side dishes.

8 SERVINGS	**15 MINS**	**4 TO 6 HOURS** + MARINATING

INGREDIENTS

1 tablespoon (7 g/0.2 oz) onion powder

1 tablespoon (9 g/0.3 oz) garlic powder

1 teaspoon ground cumin

1 teaspoon ground cinnamon

1 teaspoon smoked paprika

1 tablespoon (18 g/0.6 oz) salt

3½ pounds (1.6 kg) pork suitable for slow cooking, such as shoulder

½ cup (120 ml/4.1 fl oz) water

NUTRITION FACTS PER SERVING

Total carbs: 2.1 g

Fiber: 0.6 g

Net carbs: 1.5 g

Protein: 34.8 g

Fat: 36.1 g

Energy: 481 kcal

Macronutrient ratio:
Calories from carbs (1%), protein (30%), fat (69%)

You can use any pork suitable for slow cooking, such as shoulder. Mix all the spices in a bowl. Rub the spices and salt into the pork and wrap in plastic wrap. Place in the fridge for at least 4 hours or up to 3 days.

Remove from the fridge and unwrap the pork. Put it in a slow cooker, add the water, and cook for 8 to 10 hours on low or 4 to 6 hours on high until tender.

Transfer the roast to a cutting board. Discard all the liquid in the slow cooker—it's too spicy and salty to use for anything else. Place the entire roast back in the slow cooker and pull the meat apart by tearing it into shreds with two forks.

Serve immediately or let cool, transfer into an airtight container, and store in the fridge for up to 5 days.

If you don't have a slow cooker, use a regular deep, heavy-bottomed casserole dish and cook in an oven preheated to 300°F (150°C, or gas mark 2) for 4 to 6 hours.

PIGS IN A BLANKET

Are you nostalgic for the classic cocktail snack? Try my low-carb version! Serve with homemade mustard, ketchup, or BBQ sauce.

5 SERVINGS	25 MINS	1 HOUR

INGREDIENTS

2 ½ cups (250 g/8.8 oz) almond flour

¼ cup (30 g/1.1 oz) coconut flour

1 large egg

2 tablespoons (30 g/1.1 oz) softened (not melted) butter or ghee

1 teaspoon onion powder

½ teaspoon garlic powder

½ teaspoon salt

⅓ cup (30 g/1.1 oz) grated Parmesan cheese, or more almond flour

30 mini-sausages (420 g/ 14.8 oz), or regular sausages cut into small pieces

NUTRITION FACTS PER SERVING

Total carbs: 12.8 g

Fiber: 6.5 g

Net carbs: 6.3 g

Protein: 29.2 g

Fat: 49.5 g

Energy: 593 kcal

Macronutrient ratio: Calories from carbs (4%), protein (20%), fat (76%)

Preheat the oven to 350°F (175°C, or gas mark 4). Mix the almond and coconut flour, egg, and softened butter. Add the onion and garlic powder and season with salt. Add the grated Parmesan cheese and mix well. Flatten the dough slightly and place in the freezer for 15 to 20 minutes; this will make the rolling easier.

Remove from the freezer and divide the dough into equal parts based on the number of servings. Using a rolling tool, create small flat ovals. Wrap the pieces of dough around the sausages and place on a baking sheet lined with parchment paper.

Bake for about 20 minutes until the crust is light golden. When done, remove from the oven, let the pigs rest for about 10 minutes, and then serve with Ketchup (page 29), Dijon Mustard (page 31), or Spicy Chocolate BBQ Sauce (page 34).

BEST KETO ENCHILADAS

A low-carb alternative to green-sauce enchiladas, this is one of my best recipes—and it's a personal favorite, too.

 4 SERVINGS | **15 MINS** | **40 MINS**

INGREDIENTS

1 serving Chimichurri
(page 158)

2 servings Perfectly Pulled
Pork (page 163)

2 servings (4 medium)
Essential Keto Crepes
(page 24)

1 large (200 g/7.1 oz) avocado

2 jalapeño peppers, deseeded
(30 g/1.1 oz)

1 tablespoon (1 g/0.04 oz)
chopped cilantro

¼ cup (60 g/2.1 oz) sour cream

2 tablespoons (30 ml/1 fl oz) lime
juice

½ teaspoon salt

Freshly ground black pepper

½ cup (60 g/2.1 oz) shredded
hard cheese, such as manchego

NUTRITION FACTS PER SERVING

Total carbs: 9.4 g

Fiber: 5.1 g

Net carbs: 4.3 g

Protein: 25.3 g

Fat: 43.8 g

Energy: 528 kcal

Macronutrient ratio:
Calories from carbs (3%),
protein (20%), fat (77%)

Making the crepes takes just a few minutes, but the slow-cooked meat takes hours, so plan accordingly. Instead of pulled pork, you can use any slow-cooked meat: beef, pork, lamb, or even chicken!

Preheat the oven to 350°F (175°C, or gas mark 4).

Prepare the chimichurri. Make sure you have the crepes ready.

Halve, pit, and peel the avocado. Wash, halve, and deseed the jalapeños. In a bowl, combine half of the avocado, chimichurri, jalapeños, cilantro, sour cream, and lime juice and season with salt and black pepper.

Spread about a third of the avocado sauce over the bottom of a medium casserole dish (about 10 × 7 inches/25 × 18 cm).

Dice the remaining avocado and mix with another third of the avocado sauce and the pulled pork. This will be the filling for your crepes. Top each crepe with an equal amount of the filling and roll it up tightly.

Fold the crepes one by one in the casserole dish and top with the remaining avocado sauce. Sprinkle with shredded cheese. Cook in the oven for about 25 minutes. When done, let it cool for a few minutes and then serve and enjoy!

PORK SKEWERS
WITH ASPARAGUS AND ORANGE MAYO

Crowned with a zesty, homemade orange mayonnaise, tender, herb-marinated pork skewers take center stage in this low-carb dish.

4 SERVINGS	15 MINS	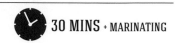 30 MINS + MARINATING

INGREDIENTS

Pork Skewers

1.3 pounds (600 g) pork, fatty shoulder

1 cup (240 ml/8 fl oz) extra virgin olive oil or ghee, melted

2 cloves garlic, crushed

1 tablespoon (4 g/0.1 oz) chopped fresh oregano

1 tablespoon (2 g/0.07 oz) chopped fresh rosemary

2 tablespoons (30 ml/1 fl oz) lemon juice

½ teaspoon salt

Pinch cayenne pepper

½ medium (100 g/3.5 oz) Spanish chorizo or salami

4 large bunches (600 g/21.2 oz) asparagus

Orange Mayo

⅓ cup (70 g/2.5 oz) Mayonnaise (page 28)

1 teaspoon freshly grated orange zest

1 tablespoon (15 ml/0.5 fl oz) fresh orange juice or lemon juice

Salt and cayenne pepper, to taste

Dice the pork into big square cubes. Set it in a medium bowl and pour the olive oil over it. Add the crushed garlic, chopped herbs, lemon juice, salt, and cayenne pepper.

Mix all the ingredients together and make sure the meat is well-coated in the oil. Set aside a small amount of oil for the asparagus. Let it rest in the fridge for 8 to 12 hours or overnight.

Meanwhile, prepare the mayo by mixing the regular mayo with the orange zest and juice, salt, and cayenne pepper. Cover with aluminum foil or place in an airtight container and refrigerate overnight.

When the meat is ready to be cooked, set the oven to broil (500°F [260°C, or gas mark 10]).

Slice the chorizo into small pieces. Pierce the skewers through each meat cube and chorizo slice. Repeat for the remaining pork pieces and chorizo.

Set the skewers on a rack and place in the oven. Cook for 10 minutes, turn, and cook for another 5 minutes. When the meat is ready, transfer the skewers to a serving plate.

Wash the asparagus and trim the woody ends. Drizzle with oil and season with salt and black pepper. Pierce batches of asparagus through two sets of skewers or place them in a baking dish. Cook in the oven for 5 to 7 minutes. When ready, the asparagus should be tender and slightly browned, yet still crisp.

Serve the asparagus hot with the pork skewers and orange mayo.

NUTRITION FACTS PER SERVING

Total carbs: 8.5 g	**Protein:** 35.5 g	**Macronutrient ratio:** Calories from carbs (3%), protein (22%), fat (75%)
Fiber: 3.6 g	**Fat:** 54.7 g	
Net carbs: 4.9 g	**Energy:** 666 kcal	

LAMB VINDALOO

If you're a spice fiend, you'll love this healthier version of the legendary Indian dish.

 4 SERVINGS | **20 MINS** | **1 HOUR 30 MINS**

INGREDIENTS

Lamb

1 small (70 g/2.5 oz) white onion

2 cloves garlic, crushed

1 to 2 small hot chile peppers

1 tablespoon (8 g/0.3 oz) grated ginger

1 bunch cilantro

1.7 pounds (800 g) lamb shoulder, boneless

2 tablespoons (30 g/1.1 oz) butter or ghee

1 teaspoon ground turmeric

1 teaspoon salt

1 small can (200 g/7.1 oz) diced tomatoes

1 tablespoon (15 ml/0.5 fl oz) balsamic vinegar

1 ½ cups (480 ml/12 fl oz) water

Freshly ground black pepper

Optional: 1 cup (230 g/8 oz) full-fat yogurt or sour cream to serve on top

Spices to Toast

1 teaspoon coriander seeds

1 teaspoon fennel seeds

1 teaspoon fenugreek seeds

2 whole cloves

¼ teaspoon whole black peppercorns

2 cloves

Peel and finely dice the onion and peel and crush the garlic. Wash, halve, and deseed the chile pepper and grate the ginger. Wash the cilantro, separate the stalks from the leaves, and finely chop the stalks. Keep the remaining leaves for garnish. Dice the lamb into medium pieces and set aside.

In a dry, hot pan, toast all of the spices for a few minutes until golden. Be careful not to let them burn.

Grease a large heavy pot or Dutch oven with ghee and add the sliced onion, garlic, chiles, ginger, and cilantro stalks. Cook over a medium heat for about 5 minutes or until the onion starts to brown.

Add the lamb, toasted spices, turmeric, salt, and black pepper. Mix well and let the meat brown on all sides. Add the chopped tomatoes, balsamic vinegar, and water. Turn the heat down, cover with a lid, and cook on medium-low for about an hour or until the meat is tender.

Check the pot every 20 minutes to ensure there is enough water and that the vindaloo isn't sticking to the bottom. When done, take off of the heat and let it sit for a few minutes. Season with more salt if needed and serve with plain Cauli-Rice (page 37) or Spicy Asian Cauli-Rice (page 189).

NUTRITION FACTS PER SERVING

Total carbs: 7.1 g   **Protein:** 37 g   **Macronutrient ratio:**
Fiber: 1.8 g   **Fat:** 41.9 g   Calories from carbs (4%), protein (27%),
Net carbs: 5.2 g   **Energy:** 559 kcal   fat (69%)

SLOW-ROAST PORK BELLY
WITH QUICK "POTATO" SALAD

High in fat, pork belly is perfect for a low-carb diet. In this recipe, it's infused with fragrant herbs and served with a satisfying cauliflower salad.

 4 SERVINGS | **25 MINS** | **2 HOURS 45 MINS** + MARINATING

INGREDIENTS

Pork Belly

1.1 pounds (500 g) pork belly

1 teaspoon fennel seeds

2 cloves garlic, crushed

2 tablespoons (5 g/0.2 oz) fresh thyme leaves

½ teaspoon salt

Freshly ground black pepper

"Potato" Salad

1 medium (600 g/21.2 oz) cauliflower

2 cups water

2 slices (30 g/1.1 oz) of thinly-cut bacon

1 pickle (65 g/2.3 oz)

2 tablespoons (6 g/0.2 oz) chopped chives or spring onion

1 tablespoon (15 ml/0.5 fl oz) lemon juice

2 tablespoons (30 g/1.1 oz) Mayonnaise (page 28)

¼ cup (60 g/2.1 oz) sour cream or more mayo

½ teaspoon salt

Freshly ground black pepper

(continued)

Preheat the oven to 400°F (200°C, or gas mark 6). Using a sharp knife, score the pork skin down to the meat. Make the cuts close together and try not to cut the meat.

Put the fennel seeds into a hot, dry pan and toast until fragrant, about 1 to 2 minutes. Mix the fennel seeds with the garlic, fresh thyme, salt, and black pepper. Rub the spices into the skin and meat. If you have time, let it marinate in the fridge overnight.

Place the pork belly in a casserole dish and cook for 30 minutes. Then, turn the heat down to 325°F (160°C, or gas mark 3) and cook for another 90 minutes. Finally, increase the temperature to 425°F (220°C, or gas mark 7) and cook for another 15 to 20 minutes. When done, remove from the oven and set it aside. Let it rest for 20 minutes before serving.

To prepare the salad, wash and quarter the cauliflower and place in a steaming rack inside a pot filled with the water. Bring to a boil and cook until tender, about 10 to 15 minutes. Drain the cauliflower, let it cool, and then chop it into small, bite-sized pieces. Transfer to a mixing bowl. Pan-fry the bacon until crispy, chop it into small pieces, and add to the bowl.

Prepare the dressing. Dice or grate the pickle into in a small bowl. Add the chives, lemon juice, mayo, and sour cream. Season with salt and black pepper to taste and add to the bowl with the cauliflower and bacon. The salad can be served warm but is best when refrigerated overnight.

When the meat is done, pour the sauce from the casserole dish into a pot and add ½ to 1 cup (120 to 240 ml/4.1 to 8.1 fl oz) of vegetable stock or broth. Add the celery, onion, garlic, and tomato puree and bring to a boil. Simmer until the gravy has reduced by half and remove from heat. Using a hand blender, pulse until smooth. Pour the gravy over the pork belly and serve with the salad.

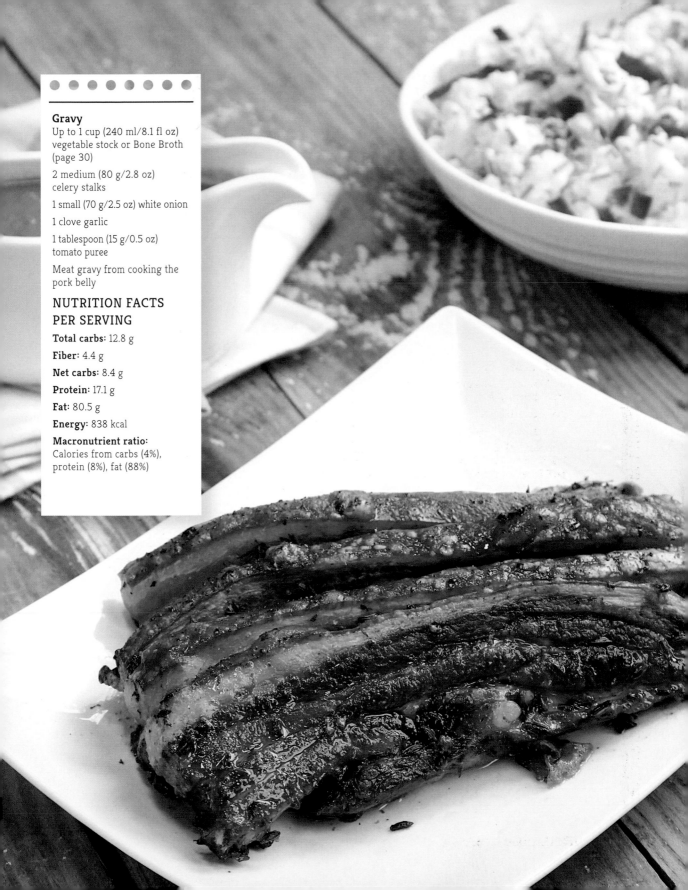

Gravy

Up to 1 cup (240 ml/8.1 fl oz) vegetable stock or Bone Broth (page 30)

2 medium (80 g/2.8 oz) celery stalks

1 small (70 g/2.5 oz) white onion

1 clove garlic

1 tablespoon (15 g/0.5 oz) tomato puree

Meat gravy from cooking the pork belly

NUTRITION FACTS PER SERVING

Total carbs: 12.8 g

Fiber: 4.4 g

Net carbs: 8.4 g

Protein: 17.1 g

Fat: 80.5 g

Energy: 838 kcal

Macronutrient ratio: Calories from carbs (4%), protein (8%), fat (88%)

DANISH MEATBALLS WITH TOMATO SAUCE

Meatballs are a staple of Danish cuisine. These are served with red sauce, and they're excellent with regular or flavored Cauli-Rice (page 37 or 189).

12 MEATBALLS	20 MINS	40 MINS

INGREDIENTS

Meatballs

2 tablespoons (30 g/1.1 oz) ghee or lard

1 small (70 g/2.5 oz) white onion

1.1 pounds (500 g) ground pork, 20% fat

½ cup (50 g/1.8 oz) almond flour

1 large egg

1 teaspoon dried thyme

1 teaspoon paprika

½ teaspoon salt

Freshly ground black pepper

4 cups (480 g/16.9 oz) of Cauli-Rice (page 37), to serve

(continued)

Heat a large pan greased with 1 tablespoon (15 g/0.5 oz) of the ghee and add the finely chopped onion. Cook over a medium heat until lightly browned; stir frequently to prevent burning.

Place the ground pork into a bowl. Add the caramelized onion, almond flour, egg, thyme, paprika, salt, and black pepper. Mix until well combined. Using your hands, form small or medium-sized meatballs or ovals. The smaller the meatballs are, the less time they will take to cook.

Place the remaining ghee in the pan and add the meatballs. Cook for about 2 minutes on each side and turn using a fork until all the sides are browned with a slight crisp.

Reduce the heat to medium-low. Add the canned tomatoes, bay leaves, crushed garlic, broth, salt, and black pepper, and cook until the sauce is reduced by half, about 30 minutes. Remove the bay leaves. Serve immediately alongside the Cauli-Rice.

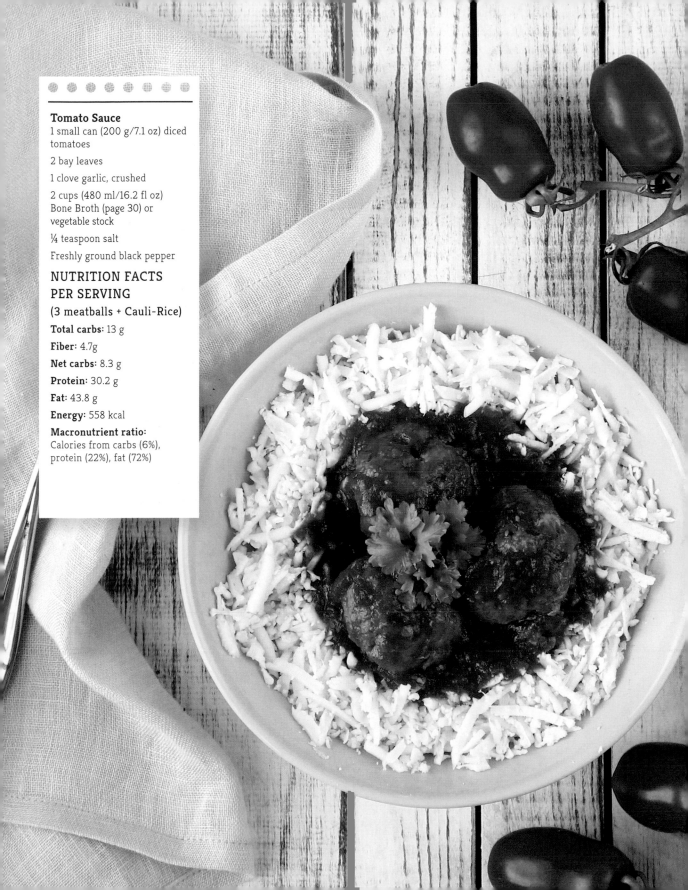

Tomato Sauce

1 small can (200 g/7.1 oz) diced tomatoes

2 bay leaves

1 clove garlic, crushed

2 cups (480 ml/16.2 fl oz) Bone Broth (page 30) or vegetable stock

¼ teaspoon salt

Freshly ground black pepper

NUTRITION FACTS PER SERVING

(3 meatballs + Cauli-Rice)

Total carbs: 13 g

Fiber: 4.7g

Net carbs: 8.3 g

Protein: 30.2 g

Fat: 43.8 g

Energy: 558 kcal

Macronutrient ratio: Calories from carbs (6%), protein (22%), fat (72%)

PORK TENDERLOIN
WITH GARLIC & KALE STUFFING

This is the ultimate pork tenderloin: roasted, juicy, and smothered in a flavorful gravy.

 8 SERVINGS | 20 MINS | 1 HOUR 20 MINS

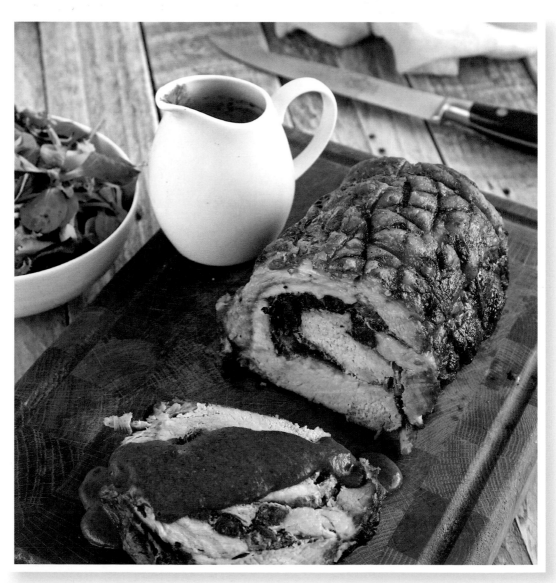

INGREDIENTS
Pork Tenderloin

1½ cups (75 g/2.6 oz) dark leaf kale (e.g. cavolo nero)

2 cups (200 g/7.1 oz) white mushrooms

2 cloves garlic, crushed

½ medium (100 g/3.5 oz) Spanish chorizo or salami

2 large eggs

3 pounds (1.4 kg) pork tenderloin, fat and skin on

1 teaspoon salt

Freshly ground black pepper

Gravy

½ cup (15 g/0.5 oz) dried wild mushrooms

Gravy from cooking the meat

2 tablespoons (30 g/1.1 oz) ghee, butter, or lard

1 cup (240 ml/8 fl oz) water, Bone Broth (page 30) or vegetable stock

1 medium (110 g/3.9 oz) white onion, chopped

1 clove garlic, crushed

NUTRITION FACTS PER SERVING
Total carbs: 4.6 g

Fiber: 1 g

Net carbs: 3.6 g

Protein: 38.3 g

Fat: 31.1 g

Energy: 514 kcal

Macronutrient ratio:
Calories from carbs (3%), protein (30%), fat (67%)

Preheat the oven to 450°F (230°C, or gas mark 8). Prepare the stuffing: Wash and chop the kale, removing any thick hard stems. Wash and slice the mushrooms. Place the crushed garlic in a hot pan greased with ghee and cook over a medium-low heat for 1 to 2 minutes.

Add the kale to the pan and cook for another 10 to 15 minutes. Add the mushrooms and diced chorizo and cook for 5 more minutes. Finally, add the eggs and cook for another 2 to 3 minutes, stirring frequently. When done, set it aside.

Prepare the tenderloin. Score the skin using a sharp knife. Make the cuts close together and cut through the skin and fat, but not through the meat.

Butterfly the tenderloin. Using a sharp knife held parallel to your work surface, start slicing the meat lengthwise, slowly pressing it out to create a flat tenderloin you can roll up. Pound it with a meat mallet if too thick. Season with salt and black pepper.

Start stuffing the tenderloin. Spread the stuffing over the meat, leaving a 1- to 2-inch (2.5 to 5 cm) border all around. Starting at a long side, roll up the pork to enclose the filling. To prevent the stuffing from falling out while roasting, fold about an inch (2.5 cm) of the short edges in as you roll. Firmly tie a kitchen string around the meat. Start by tying the loin lengthwise and then widthwise in four or five places, or place it in a butcher's netting.

Cook in the oven for 20 minutes. Turn the heat down to 325°F (160°C, or gas mark 3) and cook for another 40 minutes or until the meat thermometer reads 175°F (79°C). When done, cover with foil and let it rest while you make the gravy.

Soak the dried porcini mushrooms in 1 cup (235 ml) of water for 15 minutes and then drain. Pour the meat juices in a pan and then add the ghee, Bone Broth, chopped onion, garlic, and the mushrooms. Cook until the sauce is reduced by half and remove from the heat. Using a hand blender, pulse until smooth. If the sauce is too thick, add more water, broth, or vegetable stock.

Remove the kitchen string and slice the pork loin. Pour the gravy over the slices and serve with braised vegetables, such as Braised Cabbage with Pancetta (page 198) or Creamy Vegetable Mash (page 190).

HERB-CRUSTED RACK OF LAMB

Guaranteed to impress your guests, herb-and-macadamia-crusted rack of lamb is a great meal for special occasions, like holidays and family gatherings.

 4 SERVINGS | **15 MINS** | **30 MINS**

INGREDIENTS

2 large 8-rib racks of lamb (1.5 kg/3.3 lb)

½ teaspoon salt

Freshly ground black pepper, to taste

½ cup (65 g/2.3 oz) macadamia nuts or blanched almonds

1 tablespoon (15 g/0.5 oz) Dijon Mustard (page 31)

1 tablespoon (2 g/0.07 oz) chopped fresh rosemary leaves

¼ cup (15 g/0.5 oz) chopped fresh parsley

1 tablespoon (2 g/0.07 oz) chopped fresh thyme leaves

1 tablespoon (6 g/0.2 oz) lemon zest

2 cloves garlic

2 tablespoons (30 g/1.1 oz) ghee

NUTRITION FACTS PER SERVING

Total carbs: 3.6 g

Fiber: 2 g

Net carbs: 1.6 g

Protein: 30.4 g

Fat: 77.6 g

Energy: 834 kcal

Macronutrient ratio: Calories from carbs (1%), protein (14%), fat (85%)

Preheat the oven to 400°F (200°C, or gas mark 6). Remove the lamb from the fridge and let it sit for a few minutes at room temperature. Wash and pat dry the rack and season with salt and black pepper.

Place the macadamia nuts, mustard, rosemary, parsley, thyme, lemon zest, and garlic into a blender and pulse until smooth; or, leave a slightly crumbly texture, if you like. Season with salt and black pepper. This will form the nut-and-herb crust.

Heat a large ovenproof pan greased with ghee over a high heat. Add the lamb racks with the fatty large side down and cook for 2 to 3 minutes until browned. Turn the racks and cook on the other side for 30 seconds and then cook them standing up for another 30 seconds to seal the meat from all sides.

Transfer to a plate to cool to room temperature. Next, cover the fatty part with the nut-and-herb crust and press it in using your fingers so it won't fall off during baking.

Set the racks on a baking sheet with the crusted side up. Bake for 15 to 18 minutes (medium-rare) or 20 to 23 minutes (medium). Remove from the oven and cover with aluminum foil to rest for 10 minutes. As with steak, the meat will continue cooking from the residual heat. When done, the meat inside should be evenly cooked, pink, and juicy.

When ready to serve, use a sharp knife and gently slice each cutlet to prevent the crust from falling off.

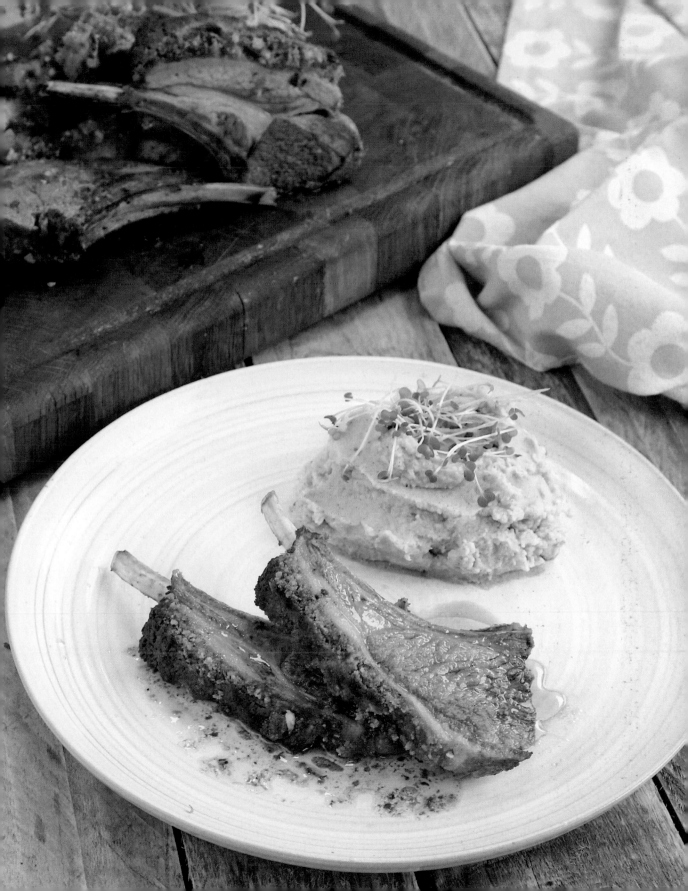

ONE-POT PORK CURRY

A zingy pork curry slow-cooked with turnips and zucchini is a stress-free, keto-friendly way to satisfy a hungry crowd.

6 SERVINGS	20 MINS	2 TO 6 HOURS

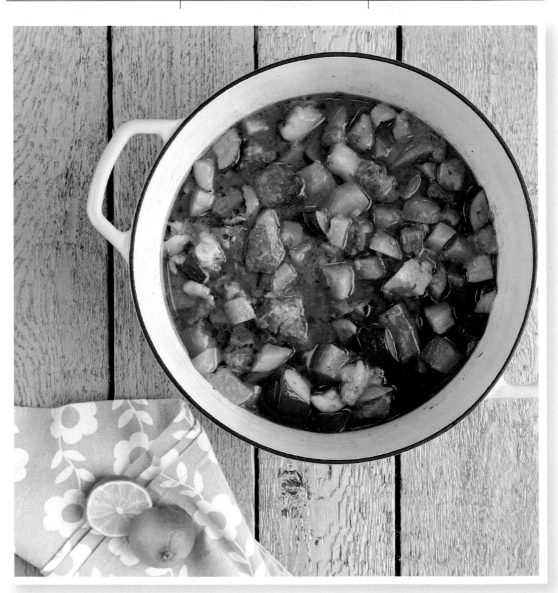

INGREDIENTS

2 tablespoons (30 g/1.1 oz) ghee or coconut oil

2 cloves garlic, crushed

1 stalk lemongrass or 1 tablespoon (6 g/0.2 oz) freshly grated lime zest

1 small (70 g/2.5 oz) white onion

2 teaspoons ginger

1 Thai chile pepper or jalapeño pepper (15 g/0.5 oz), finely chopped

1.76 pounds (800 g) pork shoulder

1 teaspoon ground cumin

½ teaspoon coriander seeds

1 teaspoon paprika

1 teaspoon salt

Freshly ground black pepper

2 limes, halved

1½ cups (360 ml/12 fl oz) coconut milk or heavy whipping cream

2 medium (400 g/14.1 oz) zucchini

2 small (300 g/10.6 oz) turnips

NUTRITION FACTS PER SERVING

Total carbs: 10.3 g

Fiber: 2.1 g

Net carbs: 8.2 g

Protein: 25.7 g

Fat: 41.5 g

Energy: 510 kcal

Macronutrient ratio: Calories from carbs (7%), protein (20%), fat (73%)

Dice the pork into medium-sized pieces and set aside. You can make the casserole in a Dutch oven, an ovenproof heavy soup pot, or in a slow cooker.

If using a Dutch oven or a heavy soup pot: Grease the pot with ghee and add the crushed garlic, lemongrass, onion, ginger, and chile pepper. Cook over a medium-high for a few minutes until the onion is golden brown.

Add the pork and brown on all sides by cooking for about 5 minutes and stirring frequently. Add all the spices. Squeeze in the lime juice and toss the four lime halves into the pot. (These are used only to infuse the curry and will be removed when it's done.) Pour in the coconut milk, lower the heat to minimum, and cover with a lid. Cook for 1½ to 2 hours or until the pork is tender.

Meanwhile, wash and dice the zucchini. Peel and dice the turnip into medium pieces. Add to the Dutch oven for the last 45 to 60 minutes of the cooking process.

If using a slow cooker: In a large pot greased with ghee, brown the garlic, onion, ginger, chile pepper, and pork pieces. Add all the spices, lemongrass, and lime halves and transfer to the slow cooker. Pour in the coconut milk and cook for 6 hours on high or for 10 hours on low. Add the turnip and zucchini for the last 2 to 3 hours of the cooking process. If you're using cream instead of coconut milk, add it in the last 30 minutes of the cooking process to prevent it from breaking.

When done cooking, remove the lime halves. Let the curry cool slightly before serving. Once cool, you can freeze it in batches for up to three months.

SHEPHERD'S PIE

Delicious British comfort food with a topping made from creamy
cauliflower instead of potato: You won't believe it's low-carb!

 6 SERVINGS | 20 MINS | 1 HOUR 15 MINS

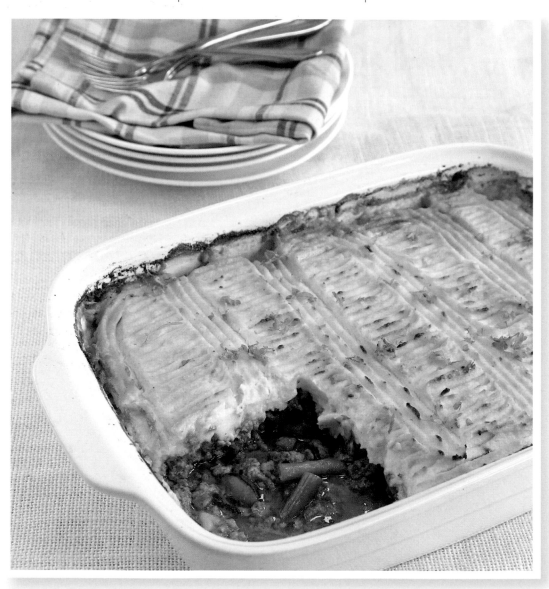

INGREDIENTS

2.2 pounds (1 kg) lamb, ground

1 small (70 g/2.5 oz) white onion

1 medium (80 g/2.8 oz) carrot

2 cloves garlic, crushed

1½ cups (150 g/5.3 oz) white mushrooms

2 cups (200 g/7.1 oz) green beans

½ cup (120 ml/4 fl oz) Bone Broth (page 30) or vegetable stock

1 tablespoon (15 ml/0.5 fl oz) Worcestershire sauce

2 tablespoons (16 g/0.6 oz) ground chia seeds

1 large (800 g/28.2 oz) cauliflower

2 tablespoons (30 g/1.1 oz) butter or ghee

1 teaspoon salt

Freshly ground black pepper

2 tablespoons (6 g/0.2 oz) chopped chives or fresh parsley

NUTRITION FACTS PER SERVING

Total carbs: 13.9 g

Fiber: 5.3 g

Net carbs: 8.6 g

Protein: 33.7 g

Fat: 40 g

Energy: 537 kcal

Macronutrient ratio: Calories from carbs (6%), protein (26%), fat (68%)

Heat a large pan and add the ground lamb. Brown from all sides, stirring frequently, until the fat is released and there are no pink parts. Use a slotted spoon to transfer the lamb to a bowl and set aside. Keep the cooking fat in the pan.

Peel and finely dice the onion and carrot and then peel and crush the garlic. Wash and slice the mushrooms. Wash and trim the green beans and chop them into quarters. Place the onion and garlic in the pan where you cooked the lamb. Cook for about 2 minutes or until translucent, stirring frequently. Add the carrot, mushrooms, and green beans. Cook for a few more minutes until the carrot begins to soften.

Return the cooked lamb to the pan and add the Bone Broth and Worcestershire sauce. Season with salt and black pepper to taste and simmer over a low heat for 20 to 25 minutes. When done, take it off of the heat and add the ground chia seeds. Mix until well combined.

Meanwhile, preheat the oven to 400°F (200°C, or gas mark 6) and prepare the cauliflower mash. Wash the cauliflower and cut it into medium florets. Place it on a steaming rack in a steaming pot filled with about 2 inches (5 cm) of water and cook for about 10 minutes.

When done, transfer the cauliflower to a blender and pulse until smooth and creamy. Add the ghee, season with salt and black pepper, and pulse again. When done, set it aside.

Spread the lamb mixture into a casserole dish. Top with mashed cauliflower. Using the tines of a fork, create a decorative pattern on top. Cook for about 30 minutes in the oven until the cauliflower is golden in color. When done, remove from the oven and let it cool slightly before serving. Top with chopped chives or parsley.

LAMB AVGOLEMONO

*Thankfully, lamb chops take less time to cook than other cuts of lamb.
Try them with a delicious Greek-style avgolemono, or egg and lemon, sauce!*

 4 SERVINGS | **15 MINS** | 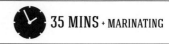 **35 MINS + MARINATING**

INGREDIENTS

Lamb

8 small lamb chops (800 g/1.76 lb)

¼ cup (60 ml/2 fl oz) olive oil

2 tablespoons (15 ml/0.5 fl oz) red or white wine vinegar

4 cloves garlic, crushed

1 tablespoon (3 g/0.1 oz) dried oregano

1 tablespoon (15 g/0.5 oz) Dijon Mustard (page 31)

1 teaspoon lemon zest

Salt and freshly ground black pepper, to taste

Avgolemono Sauce

1 cup (240 ml/8.1 fl oz) chicken stock or Bone Broth (page 30)

4 large egg yolks

½ cup (120 ml/4 fl oz) fresh lemon juice

2 tablespoons (3 g/0.1 oz) chopped chives

Salt and freshly ground black pepper, to taste

First, marinate the lamb. Set the lamb chops into a bowl that you can fit in the fridge. Mix together the oil, vinegar, crushed garlic, herbs, Dijon mustard, lemon zest, salt, and black pepper and coat the lamb on all sides with the marinade. Cover the bowl with aluminum foil and place in the fridge for at least 2 hours or overnight. Remove the lamb chops from the fridge and keep at room temperature before cooking.

Preheat the oven to 400°F (200°C, or gas mark 6). Place the chops on a baking sheet and transfer to the oven. Discard the remaining marinade. Cook for 20 to 30 minutes, depending on how well-done you like them. Turn them halfway through the cooking process so they brown evenly.

Prepare the avgolemono sauce. Pour the Bone Broth in a small pot and bring to a simmer over low heat. Meanwhile, crack the eggs and separate the egg white from the egg yolks. Reserve the whites for use in another recipe.

In a large bowl, whisk the egg yolks until frothy. Squeeze in the lemon juice and whisk until well combined. Pour two ladles of the Bone Broth, one at a time, into the bowl and keep whisking. Then, slowly pour the egg-and-lemon mixture into the simmering pot of Bone Broth and keep stirring to avoid clumping. Continue whisking until the sauce thickens and then remove from the heat. Season with salt and black pepper to taste. Add the chives and mix well. Top the chops with the sauce and serve immediately.

NUTRITION FACTS PER SERVING

Total carbs: 4.5 g | **Protein:** 41.2 g | **Macronutrient ratio:**
Fiber: 0.9 g | **Fat:** 38.1 g | Calories from carbs (3%), protein (31%),
Net carbs: 3.6 g | **Energy:** 534 kcal | fat (66%)

GREEK ROAST LAMB

This Greek-style roast makes for deliciously tender meat that falls apart at the lightest touch.

 6 SERVINGS | **15 MINS** | **3 HOURS**

INGREDIENTS

Roast Lamb

2 tablespoons each of fresh oregano, mint, and thyme, chopped

3 cloves garlic, crushed

1 tablespoon (6 g/0.2 oz) lemon zest

4.4 pounds (2 kg) lamb leg or shoulder, bone in

3 tablespoons (45 g/1.6 oz) butter or ghee

Salt and freshly ground black pepper, to taste

½ to 1 cup (120 to 240 ml/ 4.1 to 8.1 fl oz) vegetable stock or water

Tomato Sauce

Juices from cooking the lamb

1 large tin (400 g/14.1 oz) chopped tomatoes

1 clove garlic, crushed

½ cup (50 g/1.8 oz) olives

2 tablespoons (17 g/0.6 oz) capers

Salt, pepper and fresh oregano, to taste

Preheat the oven to 400°F (200°C, or gas mark 6). Mix together the freshly chopped herbs, garlic, and lemon zest. Rub the lamb with ghee and season with salt and black pepper. Using a sharp knife, create small cuts in the leg. Rub the leg with the herbs and squeeze some of it in the cuts.

Place the leg in a casserole dish, add the water or vegetable stock, cover with aluminum foil or a lid, and put in the oven. Cook for 1 hour and 45 minutes.

Increase the temperature to 375°F (190°C, or gas mark 5) and take the lid off. Cook for another 45 minutes until golden and crispy. When done, the meat should be fork-tender. Remove from the oven, place aluminum foil on top, and set aside to cool slightly.

For the sauce, pour the pan gravy into a pot and add the chopped tomatoes, crushed garlic, olives, capers, and oregano. Bring to a boil, simmer until reduced by half, and remove from the heat. Season with salt to taste. Pair with Creamy Vegetable Mash (page 190) or Braised Cabbage with Pancetta (page 198) and serve with the sauce on the side.

NUTRITION FACTS PER SERVING

Total carbs: 4.8 g   **Protein:** 31.4 g

Fiber: 1.6 g   **Fat:** 36 g

Net carbs: 3.2 g   **Energy:** 475 kcal

Macronutrient ratio: Calories from carbs (3%), protein (27%), fat (70%)

LAMB MEATBALLS WITH FETA

Feta cheese adds a salty, savory kick to these lamb meatballs and makes the sauce smooth and creamy, too. Eat with zucchini noodles—zoodles—or Cauli-Rice.

16 MEATBALLS	20 MINS	35 MINS

INGREDIENTS

Lamb Meatballs
1.1 pounds (500 g) ground lamb

1 large egg

½ cup (50 g/1.8 oz) almond flour

2 tablespoon (8 g/0.3 oz) each chopped fresh oregano and mint

1 teaspoon lemon zest

1 clove garlic, crushed

¼ cup (25 g/0.9 oz) olives

Salt and freshly ground black pepper, to taste

⅔ cup (100 g/3.5 oz) feta cheese, crumbled

1 tablespoon (15 g/0.5 oz) ghee

Zoodles
4 medium (800 g/28.2 oz) zucchini

Tomato Sauce
2 medium (120 g/4.2 oz) tomatoes, chopped

1 tablespoon (15 g/0.5 oz) unsweetened tomato puree

1 bay leaf, crumbled

1 cup (240 ml/8.1 fl oz) Bone Broth (page 30)

Salt and freshly ground black pepper, to taste

Fresh basil, for garnish

In a bowl, combine the ground lamb with the egg and almond flour. Add the chopped oregano, mint, lemon zest, garlic, and sliced kalamata or green olives. Add a pinch of salt and black pepper. Mix well and add the crumbled feta cheese. Using your hands, create medium-size meatballs and set aside.

Preheat a large pan greased with ghee. Once hot, add the meatballs and cook for about 2 to 3 minutes before turning with a fork. Cook until the outsides are browned and then add the chopped tomatoes, tomato puree, crumbled bay leaf, and Bone Broth. Season with salt and black pepper to taste.

Cook for 20 to 25 minutes on a medium-low heat and turn the meatballs halfway through the cooking process.

Meanwhile, wash the zucchini. Prepare the "zoodles" by slicing the zucchini with a julienne peeler or a vegetable spiralizer. Once the meatballs are cooked, remove them with a slotted spoon and set the zoodles into the meat and feta sauce. Cook over a medium-high heat for just 3 to 5 minutes: When done, the zoodles should still be al dente.

Alternatively, you can cook the zoodles in a separate pan greased with ghee. (Always make the zoodles just before serving and cook them briefly to avoid having them become mushy.) Serve with the meatballs and garnish with fresh basil leaves.

NUTRITION FACTS PER SERVING (4 meatballs + zoodles)

Total carbs: 12.6 g	**Protein:** 33.1 g	**Macronutrient ratio:** Calories from carbs (6%), protein (23%), fat (71%)
Fiber: 4.3 g	**Fat:** 45.8 g	
Net carbs: 8.2 g	**Energy:** 581 kcal	

MINCED PORK PIES

These savory minced pork pies are deliciously crispy,
grain-free, and so low in carbs!

 8 PIES | 20 MINS | 50 MINS

INGREDIENTS

Crust
1 cup (100 g/3.5 oz) almond flour or flax meal

2 cups (100 g/3.5 oz) ground pork rinds

¼ cup (40 g/1.4 oz) flax meal

2 large eggs

½ teaspoon salt or to taste

Filling
6 slices (90 g/3.2 oz) of thinly-cut bacon

1 tablespoon (15 g/0.5 oz) ghee or lard

10.6 ounces (300 g) ground pork, 20% fat

1 small (70 g/2.5 oz) white onion

2 cloves garlic, crushed

¾ cup (100 g/3.5 oz) cheddar cheese, grated

3.5 oz (100 g) cream cheese or soft goat cheese

2 large eggs

¼ cup (12 g/0.4 oz) chopped chives or spring onions

½ teaspoon salt

Freshly ground black pepper

Preheat the oven to 400°F (200°C, or gas mark 6). In a bowl, mix the ingredients for the crust and combine well using your hands. Add a tablespoon (15 ml/0.5 fl oz) or two of water if needed. If using salted pork rinds, omit additional salt.

Divide the batter into eight equal parts and press them into greased nonstick tart pans (ideally, you should use mini-pie pans with removable bottoms). Press the dough with your fingers toward the edges and up the sides to create a "bowl" shape.

Place the pies on a baking sheet and top with sheets of parchment paper and ceramic baking beans. Transfer to the preheated oven and bake for about 12 to 15 minutes. When done, remove from the oven and set aside.

To prepare the filling, slice the bacon and cook in a pan greased with ghee until crispy. Add the ground pork and cook, stirring frequently, until completely browned. When done, use a slotted spoon to transfer the meat and bacon into a bowl and set aside.

Place the onion and garlic in the pan in which you cooked the pork and bacon. Cook for 5 to 8 minutes over a medium-high heat until lightly browned. Set it aside.

Mix the pork, bacon, caramelized onion and garlic, and remaining ingredients in a bowl.

Combine everything well and distribute evenly into the piecrusts. Return the crusts to the oven and bake for 15 to 20 minutes. Remove from the oven and then set aside to cool. Store in the fridge and serve cold or reheat if desired.

NUTRITION FACTS PER PIE

Total carbs: 5.6 g	**Protein:** 26.9 g	**Macronutrient ratio:** Calories from carbs (3%), protein (27%), fat (70%)
Fiber: 2.7 g	**Fat:** 30.7 g	
Net carbs: 2.8 g	**Energy:** 411 kcal	

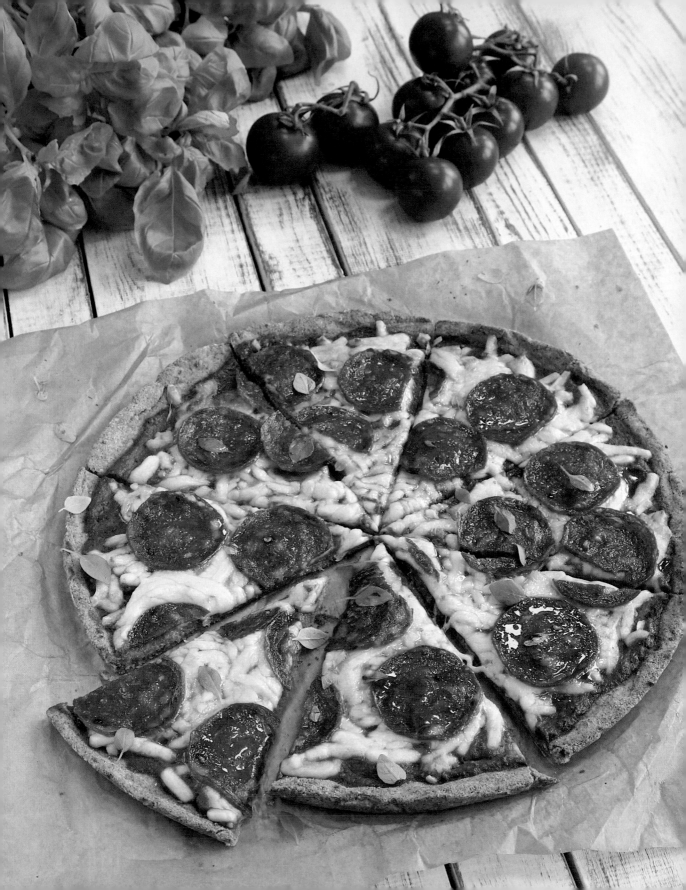

PEPPERONI PIZZA

You won't miss "real" pizza anymore:
This healthier alternative to traditional pepperoni
pizza has just a fraction of the carbs.

 4 SERVINGS | **10 MINS** | **25 MINS**

INGREDIENTS

Crust

1½ cups (150 g/5.3 oz) almond flour

¼ cup (40 g/1.4 oz) flax meal

2 tablespoons (15 g/0.5 oz) psyllium husk powder

⅓ cup (30 g/1.1 oz) grated Parmesan cheese, or more almond flour

1 teaspoon dried Italian herbs

½ teaspoon each onion powder, garlic powder and salt

1 large egg

¼ cup (60 ml/2 fl oz) lukewarm water

Topping

½ cup (120 g/4.2 oz) Marinara Sauce (page 33)

½ teaspoon chile flakes

1 cup (120 g/4.2 oz) mozzarella cheese

½ package (60 g/2.1 oz) pepperoni

2 tablespoons (5 g/0.2 oz) chopped fresh basil

1 tablespoon (15 ml/0.5 fl oz) extra virgin olive oil

Preheat the oven to 400°F (200°C, or gas mark 6). In a mixing bowl, combine the almond flour, flax meal, psyllium husk powder, grated Parmesan cheese, Italian herbs, onion and garlic powder, and salt.

Add the egg and water and combine well with your hands. Line a pizza pan or a regular large baking sheet with parchment paper. Using your hands, press the pizza dough into the pan, leaving slightly raised edges to form crusts to hold the filling. You can use a dough roller to make the surface smooth. If you don't have a pizza pan, just form the dough into a round shape. Try to make the crust as thin as possible.

Place the dough in the oven and bake for 12 to 15 minutes. When done, remove from the oven to top with the filling. Spread the marinara sauce over the dough and top with chile flakes, grated mozzarella, and pepperoni slices. Return to the oven and bake for another 10 minutes or until the cheese is melted and the pepperoni is slightly crisped up.

When done, remove the pizza from the oven and top with chopped basil and drizzle with a tablespoon (15 ml/0.5 fl oz) of extra virgin olive oil. The pizza tastes best when eaten immediately. If needed, reheat in the oven for a few minutes.

NUTRITION FACTS PER SERVING (¼ of the pizza)

Total carbs: 17 g **Protein:** 25.9 g **Macronutrient ratio:** Calories from carbs (5%), protein (18%), fat (77%)

Fiber: 9.8 g **Fat:** 47.8 g

Net carbs: 7.3 g **Energy:** 571 kcal

CREAMY MUSHROOM "RISOTTO"

This earthy mushroom risotto is a surprisingly easy, grain-free midweek meal.

6 SERVINGS	15 MINS	20 MINS

INGREDIENTS

½ cup (15 g/0.5 oz) dried porcini mushrooms

¾ cup (180 ml/6.1 fl oz) chicken stock (page 128) or vegetable stock

1 small (70 g/2.5 oz) white onion

4 cups (200 g/7.1 oz) fresh wild mushrooms

¼ cup plus 2 tablespoons (56 g/2 oz) ghee or butter

2 cloves garlic, crushed

6 cups (720 g/25.4 oz) Cauli-Rice (page 37)

Salt, to taste

½ cup (120 ml/4.1 fl oz) heavy whipping cream

1 tablespoon (15 ml/0.5 fl oz) lemon juice

¼ cup (15 g/0.5 oz) chopped fresh parsley

⅔ cup (60 g/2.1 oz) grated Parmesan cheese

Soak the dried porcinis in the chicken stock for at least 15 minutes. Once soaked, chop the mushrooms into smaller pieces if needed. Peel and finely dice the onion. Wash and slice the fresh mushrooms.

Grease a large pan or heavy soup pot with ¼ cup (60 g/2.1 oz) of ghee and add the onion and crushed garlic. Cook over a medium-high heat for 5 to 8 minutes until lightly browned.

Add the Cauli-Rice and sliced mushrooms and mix well. Pour in the soaked mushrooms with their liquid and season with salt. (You can substitute ¼ cup [60 ml/2 fl oz] of the stock with ¼ cup [60 ml/2 fl oz] dry white wine, if you like.)

Pour in the cream and cook for 8 to 10 minutes or until the cauliflower is tender but not overcooked. Remove from the heat. Add a squeeze of lemon juice, parsley, grated Parmesan cheese, and remaining ghee or butter, and mix until well combined. Garnish with more parsley and serve immediately.

NUTRITION FACTS PER SERVING

		Macronutrient ratio:
Total carbs: 11.3 g	**Protein**: 8 g	Calories from carbs (11%), protein (11%), fat (78%)
Fiber: 3.4 g	**Fat**: 24.4 g	
Net carbs: 7.9 g	**Energy**: 287 kcal	

KETO FALAFEL

Traditionally made with chickpeas, these low-carb falafel are grain- and legume-free, and they're served with a flavorful tahini dip.

 12 FALAFEL | **15 MINS** | **45 MINS**

INGREDIENTS

Falafel

3 cups (360 g/12.7 oz) Cauli-Rice (page 37)

1 small (70 g/2.5 oz) white onion

2 cloves garlic, crushed

2 tablespoons (30 g/1.1 oz) ghee

1 large egg

¼ cup (25 g/0.9 oz) almond flour

½ cup (65 g/2.3 oz) macadamia nuts

2½ tablespoons (3 g/0.1 oz) each chopped cilantro and mint

1 teaspoon lemon zest

2 teaspoons ground cumin

1 teaspoon ground turmeric

Salt and freshly ground black pepper, to taste

Tahini Dip

1 tablespoon (15 g/0.5 oz) tahini

3 tablespoons (36 g/1.3 oz) sour cream or coconut milk

1 tablespoon (15 g/0.5 oz) Mayonnaise (page 28)

1 tablespoon (15 ml/0.5 fl oz) lemon juice

Salt and freshly ground black pepper, to taste

First, prepare the Cauli-Rice.

Preheat the oven to 400°F (200°C, or gas mark 6).

Meanwhile, peel and finely slice the onion and garlic and add to a pan greased with ghee. Cook for 5 to 8 minutes, stirring frequently, and take off the heat.

When the Cauli-Rice is cooked, transfer it to a blender and add the caramelized onion, garlic, egg, almond flour, macadamia nuts, cilantro, mint, lemon zest, cumin, turmeric, salt, and black pepper. Pulse until smooth.

Using your hands, create medium balls or patties from the mixture and place on a baking sheet lined with parchment paper. Spray or drizzle each falafel with the remaining ghee or coconut oil and transfer to the oven. Bake for 25 to 30 minutes or until golden brown.

Meanwhile, prepare the tahini dip. Mix the tahini, sour cream, mayo, and lemon juice. Season with salt and black pepper to taste. Use as dip for the falafel.

When the falafel are done, remove them from the oven. Eat warm or cold.

NUTRITION FACTS PER SERVING (3 falafel)

Total carbs: 12.6 g **Protein:** 7.4 g **Macronutrient ratio:** Calories from carbs (9%), protein (9%), fat (82%)

Fiber: 5 g **Fat:** 31.8 g

Net carbs: 7.6 g **Energy:** 346 kcal

Chapter Eight:

SIDES

When you're following a ketogenic diet, you usually have to avoid popular side dishes, like mashed potato, rice, and spaghetti, which are very high in carbohydrates. But that doesn't mean you need to feel deprived. Far from it! In this chapter, I'll show you how to make satiating side dishes using healthy, low-carb ingredients, like the wonderfully-versatile cauliflower, which can mimic rice in almost any dish. You'll also find plenty of easy-to-make recipes that focus on tasty seasonal vegetables, like zucchini fries, bacon-laden Brussels sprouts, and steamed fresh broccoli draped with a creamy blue cheese sauce. Are you hungry yet?

CAULI-RICE THREE WAYS

Cauliflower is your new best friend. Use it instead of potatoes to create a creamy cauliflower mash; substitute it for rice; or use it to make a low-carb pizza crust!

 4 SERVINGS | **15 MINS** | **20 MINS**

INGREDIENTS

5 cups (600 g/21.2 oz) Cauli-Rice (page 37)

2 cloves of garlic

2 tablespoons (30 g/1.1 oz) ghee or butter

Salt and freshly ground black pepper, to taste

Mediterranean Rice

3 to 4 tablespoons (12 to 16 g/0.4 to 0.6 oz) fresh basil, thyme leaves, and oregano

1 small (70 g /2.5 oz) white onion

1 tablespoon (15 g/0.5 oz) tomato puree, unsweetened

Creamy Lemon Rice

2 tablespoons (5 g/0.2 oz) finely chopped fresh basil

1 tablespoon each finely chopped fresh oregano and thyme leaves

1 tablespoon (6 g/0.2 oz) lemon zest

½ cup (120 ml/4.1 fl oz) coconut milk or heavy whipping cream

2 tablespoons (30 ml/1 fl oz) lemon juice

Spicy Asian Rice

1 tablespoon (8 g/0.3 oz) ginger

Small bunch cilantro, chopped, with leaves separated from stalks

1 to 2 small chile peppers,

1 teaspoon ground turmeric

For Mediterranean Cauli-Rice:

Wash and chop the herbs, peel and mash the garlic, and finely dice the onion. Heat a pan greased with ghee over medium heat and add the mashed garlic and diced onion.

Cook, stirring frequently, for about 5 minutes or until lightly browned. Add the Cauli-Rice and cook for 5 to 7 minutes, stirring constantly. Add the tomato puree and seasonings and mix well. Finally, add the chopped herbs and cook for another 2 to 3 minutes. Season with salt and black pepper and set aside. Serve with fish and meat dishes, or top with a fried egg or sliced avocado for a quick breakfast meal!

For Creamy Lemon Cauli-Rice:

Wash and finely chop the herbs. Peel and mash the garlic and zest the lemon. Heat a pan greased with ghee over medium heat and add the mashed garlic and lemon zest. Cook for about 2 minutes, stirring frequently. Add the Cauli-Rice and cook for 1 to 2 minutes, stirring frequently. Pour in the coconut milk or cream and lemon juice. Cook for another 5 minutes. Finally, add the chopped herbs and cook for 2 to 3 minutes. Season with salt and black pepper and serve.

For Spicy Asian Cauli-Rice:

Peel and mash the garlic. Heat a large pan greased with ghee or coconut oil. Add the mashed garlic, ginger, chopped cilantro stalks, and chile pepper. Cook on medium-high heat for 3 to 5 minutes, stirring frequently. Add the Cauli-Rice and cook for 5 to 7 minutes, stirring frequently. Add the turmeric and cilantro leaves and cook for another 2 to 3 minutes. Season with salt and black pepper and serve.

NUTRITION FACTS PER SERVING
Mediterranean / Creamy Lemon / Spicy Asian

Total carbs: 10.6/10.2/8.8 g

Fiber: 3.7/3.6/3.3 g

Net carbs: 6.8/6.6/5.5 g

Protein: 3.3/3.7/3.1 g

Fat: 8/19.4/8 g

Energy: 119/223/112 kcal

Macronutrient ratio:
Calories from carbs (24/12/21%), protein (12/7/12%), fat (64/81/68%)

CREAMY VEGETABLE MASH

This creamy mash made from low-carb vegetables, fresh herbs, and spices can be paired with just about any meat dish.

 6 SERVINGS | **15 MINS** | **20 MINS**

INGREDIENTS

1 large (600 g/21.2 oz) head cauliflower

1 small (200 g/7.1 oz) head broccoli

1 medium (200 g/7.1 oz) turnip

¼ cup (56 g/2 oz) ghee or butter

1 small (70 g/2.5 oz) white onion, chopped

2 cloves garlic, crushed

Salt and freshly ground black pepper, to taste

Optional: ½ cup (45 g/1.6 oz) grated Parmesan cheese, cheddar cheese, or sour cream

NUTRITION FACTS PER SERVING

Total carbs: 10.8 g

Fiber: 3.7 g

Net carbs: 7.1 g

Protein: 3.4 g

Fat: 9.6 g

Energy: 135 kcal

Macronutrient ratio:
Calories from carbs (22%), protein (10%), fat (68%)

Wash the cauliflower and broccoli and cut into smaller florets. Peel and quarter the turnip. Place the vegetables on a steaming rack inside a pot filled with about 2 inches (5 cm) of water. Bring to a boil and cook for about 10 minutes until tender—do not overcook.

Heat a pan greased with half of the ghee and add the chopped onion and garlic. Cook for about 5 to 8 minutes or until caramelized. Keep stirring to prevent burning and then remove from the heat.

Place the cooked cauliflower, broccoli, and turnip into a blender. Add the onion and garlic and the remaining ghee. Pulse until smooth and creamy. Season to taste and stir in the cheese or sour cream, if using. Serve with meat dishes. This is also a great topping for Shepherd's Pie (page 178), instead of a regular cauliflower mash.

TIP

Try using your favorite herbs and spices in this recipe. For a Mediterranean twist, add 2 to 3 tablespoons (5 to 8 g/0.2 to 0.3 oz) chopped fresh basil, thyme, and oregano. For Asian-style, add 2 tablespoons (2 g/0.1 oz) chopped fresh cilantro, 1 tablespoon (8 g/0.3 oz) ginger, and 1 small chile pepper. For a smoky BBQ taste, add 1 teaspoon smoked paprika and ¼ teaspoon cayenne pepper. For a "curried" mash, add 1 teaspoon curry powder and ½ teaspoon ground turmeric.

GRILLED MEDITERRANEAN VEGETABLES

Crispy Mediterranean-style vegetables go well with fish and poultry—and topping them with fried eggs transforms them into a quick, healthy breakfast, too.

 6 SERVINGS | **10 MINS** | **20 MINS**

INGREDIENTS

¼ cup (56 g/2 oz) ghee or butter

3 cloves garlic, crushed

2 small (200 g/7.1 oz) red, orange, or yellow peppers

3 medium (600 g/21.2 oz) zucchini

1 medium (500 g/17.6 oz) eggplant

1 medium (100 g/3.5 oz) red onion

1 tablespoon (4 g/0.2 oz) chopped fresh oregano

2 tablespoons (5 g/0.2 oz) chopped fresh basil

Salt and freshly ground black pepper, to taste

NUTRITION FACTS PER SERVING

Total carbs: 11.9 g

Fiber: 4.9 g

Net carbs: 7 g

Protein: 2.7 g

Fat: 9.8 g

Energy: 140 kcal

Macronutrient ratio: Calories from carbs (22%), protein (9%), fat (69%)

Set the oven to broil (500°F [260°C, or gas mark 10]). In a small bowl, mix the melted ghee and crushed garlic.

Wash all the vegetables. Halve, deseed, and slice the bell peppers into strips. Slice the zucchini widthwise into ¼-inch (about ½ cm) pieces. Wash the eggplant and slice. Quarter each slice into ¼-inch (about ½ cm) pieces. Peel and slice the onion into medium wedges and separate the sections using your hands. Place the vegetables into a bowl and add the chopped herbs, ghee with garlic, salt, and black pepper.

Spread all the vegetables on a baking sheet, ideally on a roasting rack or net so that the vegetables don't become soggy from the juices. Transfer to the oven and cook for about 15 minutes. Be careful not to burn them.

When done, the vegetables should be slightly tender but still crisp. Serve with meat dishes or bake with cheese such as feta, mozzarella, or halloumi.

BROCCOLI PATTIES

Make and freeze these easy broccoli patties ahead of time and then defrost as needed: they can be served hot or chilled, and they're great for breakfast as well.

15 PATTIES	10 MINS	35 MINS

INGREDIENTS

1 medium (400 g/14.1 oz) head broccoli

2 tablespoons (30 g/1.1 oz) ghee or lard

1 medium (110 g/3.9 oz) white onion, finely sliced

2 cloves garlic, crushed

3 large eggs

½ cup (60 g/2.1 oz) grated cheddar cheese or Parmesan cheese

Salt and freshly ground black pepper, to taste

NUTRITION FACTS PER SERVING

(3 patties)

Total carbs: 8.1 g

Fiber: 2.5 g

Net carbs: 5.7 g

Protein: 9.3 g

Fat: 13.2 g

Energy: 183 kcal

Macronutrient ratio: Calories from carbs (13%), protein (21%), fat (66%)

Preheat the oven to 400°F (200°C, or gas mark 6). Wash the broccoli and cut into florets. Place on a steaming rack in a steaming pot filled with about 2 inches (5 cm) of water and cook for about 5 to 7 minutes. Don't overcook the broccoli; it should still be al dente. When done, set it aside and let cool before chopping and mixing with the other ingredients.

Heat a pan greased with ghee and add the onion and crushed garlic. Cook for 5 to 8 minutes until lightly browned.

In a bowl, mix the eggs, cheese, salt, and black pepper. Cut the cooked broccoli into smaller pieces and place in the bowl with the eggs. Add the onion and garlic and mix until well combined.

Using a spoon, create 15 palm-size patties (3 per serving) and place them on a baking sheet lined with parchment paper. Transfer to the oven and cook for about 20 minutes or until the tops are lightly browned and crispy.

When done, remove from the oven and set aside to cool or serve immediately.

ZUCCHINI FRIES

Skip the French fries and reach for this potato-free version instead: these fries are made from zucchini, and covered in crispy pork rinds.

 4 SERVINGS | **10 MINS** | **30 TO 35 MINS**

INGREDIENTS

4 medium (800 g/28.2 oz) zucchini

¼ teaspoon salt

2 tablespoons (14 g/0.5 oz) flaxseed meal

1½ cups (75 g/2.6 oz) ground pork rinds

1 tablespoon (5 g/0.2 oz) dried Italian herbs (basil, thyme, oregano)

1 teaspoon garlic powder

1 teaspoon onion powder

Freshly ground black pepper, to taste

1 large egg

2 tablespoons (30 g/1.1 oz) ghee or coconut oil

Optional: ⅓ cup (30 g/1.1 oz) grated Parmesan cheese instead of ½ cup pork rinds

NUTRITION FACTS PER SERVING

Total carbs: 8.9 g

Fiber: 3.4 g

Net carbs: 5.5 g

Protein: 17.1 g

Fat: 12.8 g

Energy: 236 kcal

Macronutrient ratio:
Calories from carbs (11%), protein (33%), fat (56%)

Preheat the oven to 425°F (220°C, or gas mark 7). Wash the zucchini and cut into about ½-inch-wide (1.3 cm) and 3-inch-long (7.5 cm) "fries". Season with some of the salt and let rest on a cutting board for at least 20 minutes. Then pat the moisture off the fries with a paper towel.

Meanwhile, mix the "breading." Place the flaxseed meal into a bowl and combine with the ground pork rinds. Add the dried herbs, onion and garlic powder, a pinch of salt, and black pepper.

In a small bowl, mix the egg with another pinch of salt. Dip each zucchini piece in the egg and transfer to the bowl with the breading. Dredge the zucchini in the breading and place on a baking sheet lined with parchment paper. Do not put all the fries with the egg in the breading at once or it will clump up. Drizzle the fries with melted ghee or spray with coconut oil.

Transfer the sheet into the oven and bake for 20 to 25 minutes or until lightly browned and crispy. Remove from the oven and set aside to cool. Eat immediately or the fries will get soggy. If needed, place them in the oven to crisp up just before serving.

Serve with meat-based dishes and pair with Ketchup (page 29), Mayonnaise (page 28), or Spicy Chocolate BBQ Sauce (page 34)!

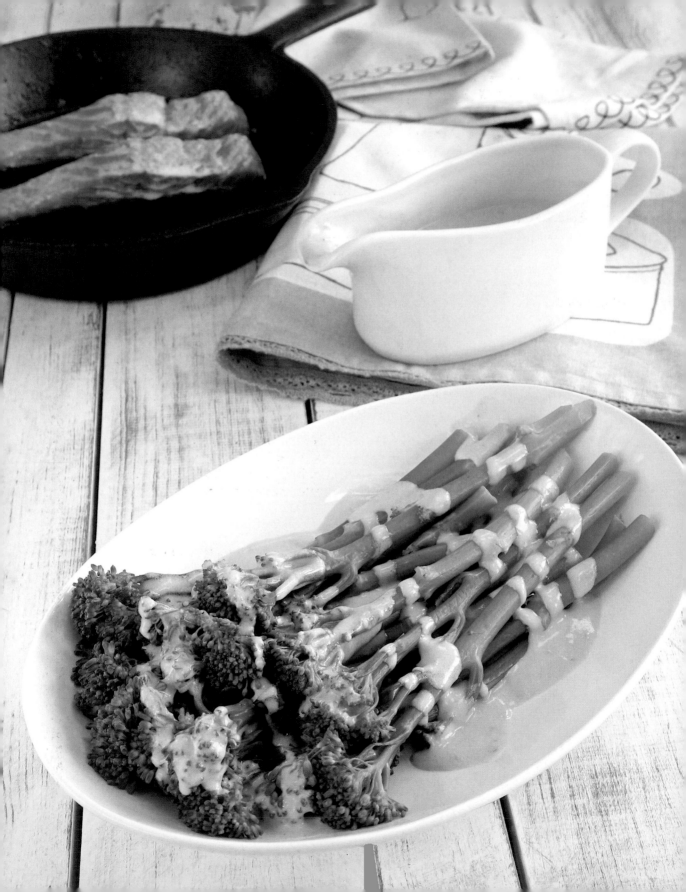

STEAMED BROCCOLI
WITH BLUE CHEESE SAUCE

Crispy broccoli and creamy blue cheese are heavenly together, and this sauce is no exception. What's more, it's fabulous with fish and seafood.

 4 SERVINGS | **10 MINS** | **15 MINS**

INGREDIENTS

1 medium (500 g/17.6 oz) head of broccoli

¼ cup (60 ml/2 fl oz) heavy whipping cream

2.1 ounces (60 g) cream cheese

2 tablespoons (30 g/1.1 oz) butter or ghee

2 ounces (56 g) crumbled blue cheese

Salt and freshly ground black pepper, to taste

NUTRITION FACTS PER SERVING

Total carbs: 9.5 g

Fiber: 3.3 g

Net carbs: 6.2 g

Protein: 8 g

Fat: 19.7 g

Energy: 231 kcal

Macronutrient ratio:
Calories from carbs (10%), protein (14%), fat (76%)

Wash the broccoli and cut into florets. Place on a steaming rack in a steaming pot filled with about 2 inches (5 cm) of water and bring to a boil. Cook for 5 to 8 minutes until the broccoli is tender but still crisp. Do not overcook. When done, set it aside.

Prepare the blue cheese sauce. Pour the cream in a small pot and add the cream cheese and butter or ghee. Gently bring to a simmer over a medium-low heat and stir until well combined and the cream cheese and butter are melted. If you need to thicken the sauce, boil for 3 to 5 more minutes, stirring frequently.

Remove from the heat and add the crumbled blue cheese. Stir until the blue cheese is dissolved and the sauce is smooth and creamy. Season with salt and black pepper, to taste. If you need to thin the sauce, add a splash of water or cream.

TIP

Try this recipe with other types of cheese: goat cheese, cheddar, or even Brie.

GARLIC-&-HERB CAULIFLOWER

Crisp, sweet, roasted cauliflower infused with fragrant herbs and spices can stand up to any meat dish imaginable.

4 SERVINGS	5 MINS	20 MINS

INGREDIENTS

1 large (800 g/28.2 oz) head cauliflower

¼ cup (56 g/2 oz) melted ghee, lard, or butter

¼ cup (10 g/0.4 oz) chopped fresh herbs (e.g., basil, oregano, and thyme)

2 tablespoons (30 ml/1 fl oz) lemon juice

3 cloves garlic, crushed

Salt and freshly ground black pepper, to taste

Optional: Parmesan for sprinkling

NUTRITION FACTS PER SERVING

Total carbs: 11.5 g

Fiber: 4.3 g

Net carbs: 7.2 g

Protein: 4.1 g

Fat: 14.4 g

Energy: 181 kcal

Macronutrient ratio: Calories from carbs (16%), protein (10%), fat (74%)

Preheat the oven to 450°F (230°C, or mark 8). Wash the cauliflower, cut into smaller florets, and place in a bowl. In another bowl, mix the melted ghee, chopped herbs, lemon juice, and crushed garlic. Season with salt and black pepper, to taste.

Add the herb mixture to the bowl with the cauliflower and coat thoroughly. Sprinkle with Parmesan cheese, if using, and place the cauliflower on a baking sheet. Transfer the sheet to the oven and bake for 15 minutes or until the cauliflower turns golden. When done, remove it from the oven and serve immediately.

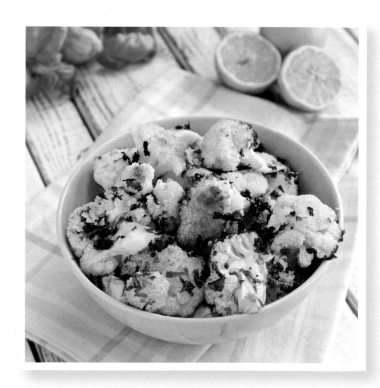

CAULI-PIZZA TARTLETS

Pizza crust made from "riced" cauliflower is remarkably tasty and works well when it's thin and crispy. Feel free to add your favorite toppings to these pizza tartlets!

 4 SERVINGS | **15 MINS** | **50 MINS**

INGREDIENTS

Pizza Crust

2 cups (240 g/8.5 oz) Cauli-Rice (page 37)

¾ cup (90 g/3.2 oz) grated mozzarella cheese

⅓ cup (30 g/1.1 oz) grated Parmesan cheese

½ teaspoon each garlic powder and onion powder

1 large egg white

2 teaspoons dried Italian herbs

1 tablespoon (15 g/0.5 oz) ghee or coconut oil

Salt and freshly ground black pepper, to taste

Topping

⅓ cup (80 g/2.8 oz) Marinara Sauce (page 33)

½ cup (50 g/1.8 oz) olives

¼ cup (30 g / 1.1 oz) grated mozzarella cheese

Fresh basil, to taste

Preheat the oven to 400°F (200°C, or gas mark 6). Prepare the Cauli-Rice and cook it in a pan or in a microwave oven. Using your hands or a cheesecloth, squeeze out as much liquid from the cauliflower as possible. Drier Cauli-Rice helps the "dough" to bind and to crisp up when baked.

In a bowl, mix the Cauli-Rice, grated mozzarella cheese, Parmesan cheese, garlic and onion powder, egg white, and Italian herbs. Season with salt and black pepper. Reserve some grated mozzarella cheese or topping.

Place the cauliflower mixture on a baking sheet lined with parchment paper and, using your hands, form four small, rounded crusts and press down to flatten. (You'll need to use firm parchment paper for this: don't substitute wax paper.) Brush or spray the crusts with some ghee or coconut oil and bake in the oven for about 20 minutes.

Remove from the oven, put another piece of parchment paper on the top of the crusts, and flip them over. Carefully peel off the top piece of parchment. Top with the marinara sauce, pitted olives, and the remaining mozzarella cheese. Return to the oven for another 10 minutes. Garnish with basil before serving.

NUTRITION FACTS PER TART

Total carbs: 7 g   **Protein:** 13.2 g

Fiber: 2.3 g   **Fat:** 18.4 g

Net carbs: 4.7 g   **Energy:** 243 kcal

Macronutrient ratio: Calories from carbs (8%), protein (22%), fat (70%)

BRAISED CABBAGE
WITH PANCETTA

Cabbage is a staple vegetable in low-carb diets. Sound boring? It's not!
Bacon and homemade Bone Broth can lift the humble cabbage to new heights.

 4 SERVINGS | **10 MINS** | **55 MINS**

INGREDIENTS

1 head (700 g/24.7 oz) green or white cabbage

1 small (70 g/2.5 oz) white onion

2 tablespoons (30 g/1.1 oz) lard, ghee, or tallow

6 slices (90 g/3.2 oz) of pancetta or thinly-cut bacon

1 cup (240 ml/8.1 fl oz) Bone Broth (page 30), chicken stock (page 128), or vegetable stock

2 tablespoons (30 ml/1 fl oz) apple cider vinegar

Salt and freshly ground black pepper, to taste

NUTRITION FACTS PER SERVING

Total carbs: 11.8 g

Fiber: 4.7 g

Net carbs: 7.1 g

Protein: 5.9 g

Fat: 14.1 g

Energy: 184 kcal

Macronutrient ratio:
Calories from carbs (16%), protein (13%), fat (71%)

Wash, halve, and slice the cabbage. Remove the hard center and discard. Peel and finely slice the onion. Grease a heavy pot or a Dutch oven with the lard and add the sliced onion and pancetta. Cook for 5 to 8 minutes, stirring frequently. Add the shredded cabbage, Bone Broth, and vinegar and mix well. Add the erythritol or liquid stevia, if using. Season with salt and black pepper to taste.

Cover with a lid and cook over a medium-low heat for 40 to 45 minutes or until tender. Keep an eye on it: add ¼ cup (60 ml/2 fl oz) of water, if needed. You don't want to have too much liquid left, but you don't want the cabbage to burn. Serve this with meat dishes, especially pork.

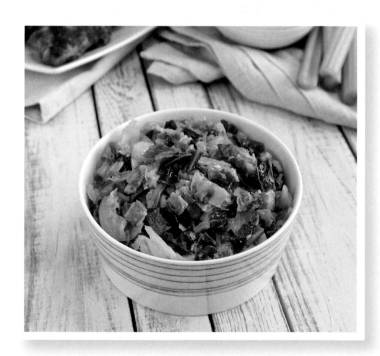

SHREDDED BRUSSELS SPROUTS
WITH BACON

Even folks who usually turn up their noses at Brussels sprouts will agree that these shredded sprouts with bacon, ghee, and lemon are ridiculously delicious.

 4 SERVINGS | **10 MINS** | **20 TO 25 MINS**

INGREDIENTS

6 cups (500 g/17.6 oz) Brussels sprouts

2 tablespoons (30 g/1.1 oz) lard, ghee, or tallow, melted

2 cloves garlic, crushed

2 tablespoons (30 ml/1 fl oz) freshly squeezed lemon juice

Salt and freshly ground black pepper, to taste

6 pieces (90 g/3.2 oz) bacon, thinly sliced

NUTRITION FACTS PER SERVING

Total carbs: 12.1 g

Fiber: 4.8 g

Net carbs: 7.3 g

Protein: 7.4 g

Fat: 13.5 g

Energy: 188 kcal

Macronutrient ratio: Calories from carbs (16%), protein (16%), fat (68%)

Preheat the oven to 400°F (200°C, or gas mark 6). Wash the Brussels sprouts and remove any dry or discolored leaves. Place in a food processor and finely slice using a slicing blade. Mix the lard with the garlic.

Spread the sprouts over a large baking sheet and drizzle with the melted lard, crushed garlic mixture, and lemon juice. Season with salt and black pepper, add the bacon, and mix until well combined.

Cook in the oven for 15 to 20 minutes, mixing twice to ensure even cooking. When done, remove from the oven and set aside for a few minutes before serving. Eat as a side or top with a fried egg for a savory, keto-friendly breakfast.

BRAISED VEGETABLES WITH TURMERIC

*Indian spices and turmeric lend fresh vegetables a bright
color and a vibrant flavor in this easy-to-prepare dish.*

 6 SERVINGS | **10 MINS** | **35 MINS**

INGREDIENTS

3 medium (600 g/21.2 oz) zucchini

1 medium (500 g/17.6 oz) eggplant

2 medium (200 g/7.1 oz) tomatoes

1 small (70 g/2.5 oz) white onion

¼ cup (56 g/2 oz) ghee, lard, or tallow

2 cloves garlic, crushed

1 teaspoon ground turmeric

½ teaspoon ground coriander seeds

½ teaspoon ground cumin seeds

¼ teaspoon ground ginger

1 star anise

½ teaspoon cinnamon

Salt and freshly ground black pepper, to taste

NUTRITION FACTS PER SERVING

Total carbs: 11.4 g

Fiber: 4.8 g

Net carbs: 6.6 g

Protein: 2.7 g

Fat: 9.9 g

Energy: 136 kcal

Macronutrient ratio:
Calories from carbs (21%), protein (8%), fat (71%)

Wash all the vegetables. Using a potato peeler or sharp knife, create wide noodles from the zucchini. Alternatively, dice it into medium-size pieces. Wash and chop the eggplant into 1-inch (2.5 cm) pieces. Chop the tomatoes. Peel and finely slice the onion.

Grease a large heavy pot or a Dutch oven with the ghee and heat over a medium-high heat. Add the onion and crushed garlic. Cook for 5 to 8 minutes until lightly browned and stir frequently to prevent burning.

Lower the heat to medium-low and add the eggplant and zucchini. Toss in all the spices, salt, and black pepper and mix well. Cover with a lid and cook for about 15 to 20 minutes. Add the chopped tomatoes and cook for another 5 to 10 minutes or until tender. When done, remove from the heat. Serve this dish with meat dishes.

SHAVED ASPARAGUS WITH PARMESAN CHEESE

This crunchy, refreshing side complements all kinds of fish and poultry. Plus, raw asparagus is high in prebiotics that improve digestion and enhance weight loss.

4 SERVINGS	**5 MINS**	**5 MINS**

INGREDIENTS

4 bunches (600 g/21.2 oz) asparagus

1⅓ cups (120 g/4.2 oz) grated or flaked Parmesan cheese

2 tablespoons (30 ml/1 fl oz) lemon juice

3 tablespoons (45 ml/1.5 fl oz) extra virgin olive oil

Salt and freshly ground black pepper, to taste

NUTRITION FACTS PER SERVING

Total carbs: 7.3 g

Fiber: 3.2 g

Net carbs: 4.1 g

Protein: 14.1 g

Fat: 18.1 g

Energy: 238 kcal

Macronutrient ratio: Calories from carbs (7%), protein (24%), fat (69%)

Wash the asparagus and slice as thinly as possible using a julienne peeler. Divide between serving plates and sprinkle with the Parmesan cheese. Drizzle with olive oil and season with salt and black pepper. Serve as a side with meat dishes.

TIP

Not a fan of raw asparagus? Bake it! Preheat the oven to 425°F (220°C, or gas mark 7). Snip the woody ends off the asparagus spears, toss with the oil and lemon juice, and season with salt and black pepper, to taste. Top with the Parmesan cheese and bake for 5 to 7 minutes.

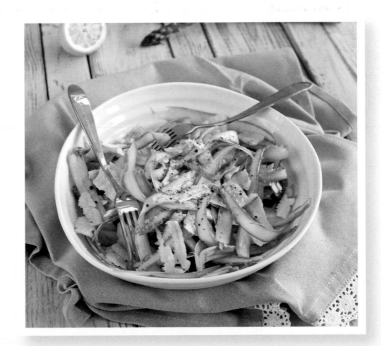

Chapter Nine:

DRINKS & DESSERTS

Finding low-carb or ketogenic drinks and desserts can be a bit of a challenge—but this chapter is here to help. When you're living a ketogenic lifestyle, you'll be spending more time preparing food, so healthy keto-friendly beverages, like breakfast smoothies, can act as quick meal replacements when you're pressed for time. And as for desserts—well, this chapter's packed with the best low-carb, grain- and sugar-free treats I've ever created, and they'll satisfy your sweet tooth every time. (Just remember that they should only be eaten once in a while!)

CREAMY KETO SMOOTHIE

Boost your energy levels with this luscious low-carb smoothie: a dose of MCT oil gives it extra fat-burning power.

1 SERVING	5 MINS	5 MINS

INGREDIENTS

½ cup (120 ml/4.1 fl oz) coconut milk or heavy whipping cream

½ cup (120 ml/4.1 fl oz) almond milk

1 tablespoon (15 g/0.5 oz) MCT oil

1 vanilla bean or 1 teaspoon unsweetened vanilla extract

¼ cup (35 g/1.2 oz) raspberries, blackberries, or strawberries, fresh or frozen

¼ cup (25 g/0.9 oz) whey protein or egg white protein powder

Few ice cubes

Optional: 3 to 5 drops liquid stevia, or 1 tablespoon (10 g/ 0.4 oz) erythritol or Swerve

Optional: 1 tablespoon (16 g/0.6 oz) macadamia nut butter or Toasted Nut Butter (page 39)

Wash the berries. Place everything into a blender and pulse until smooth. You're done! You can add a few drops of liquid stevia or erythritol if you prefer a sweeter taste. Adding nut butter will increase the fat content and will make the consistency thicker.

TIP

Medium-chain triglycerides (MCTs) are saturated fats our bodies can digest very easily. MCTs, which are mostly found in coconut oil, behave differently when ingested and are passed directly to the liver to be used as an immediate form of energy. They're also present in butter and palm oil in smaller quantities. MCTs are used by athletes to improve and enhance performance and are great for fat loss. Unlike coconut oil and butter, pure MCT oils do not solidify even when refrigerated, so they're handy for making cold smoothies.

NUTRITION FACTS PER SERVING

Total carbs: 7.5 g

Fiber: 1.2 g

Net carbs:: 6.3 g

Protein: 23.1 g

Fat: 38.6 g

Energy: 452 kcal

Macronutrient ratio: Calories from carbs (5%), protein (20%), fat (75%)

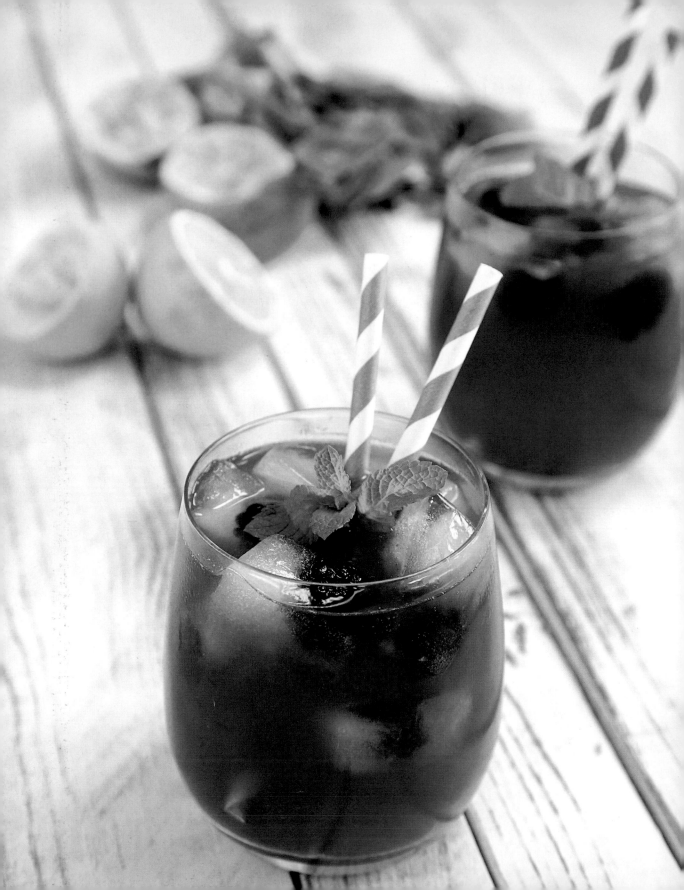

REFRESHING ICED TEA
WITH BERRY ICE CUBES

Perfect for a sultry summer afternoon, this refreshing, sugar-free drink is packed with fresh mint and served with pretty berry-laden ice cubes.

 4 SERVINGS | **5 MINS** | **2 HOURS**

INGREDIENTS

2 to 3 cups (475 to 700 ml/16 to 23.7 fl oz) hot water

4 bags quality green, white, or black tea

3 to 4 tablespoons (24 to 32 g/0.8 to 1.1 oz) ginger

2 cups fresh mint leaves

1 cup (140 g/4.9 oz) berries, such as blackberries, raspberries, strawberries, or blueberries

1 quart water, plus more for ice

½ cup (120 ml/4.1 oz) fresh lemon juice

Optional: 5 to 10 drops liquid stevia or 2 tablespoons (20 g/ 0.7 oz) erythritol or Swerve

NUTRITION FACTS PER SERVING

Total carbs: 3.9 g

Fiber: 0.5 g

Net carbs: 3.4 g

Protein: 1 g

Fat: 0.2 g

Energy: 20 kcal

Macronutrient ratio:
Calories from carbs (70%), protein (21%), fat (9%)

Pour the water over the tea bags, steep for 3 to 5 minutes, and then remove the bags and discard. Pour the tea into a large jug and add the ginger and mint. Save some mint for garnish. Let the tea rest and infuse until cooled.

Meanwhile, make the berry ice cubes. Wash the berries and put 1 to 2 small berries in each of the cube molds in an ice cube tray. Cover with water and freeze for 2 hours or until solid.

When the tea has cooled, strain it through a sieve, add the lemon juice, and refrigerate for at least an hour or until cold. Serve with the berry ice cubes and garnish with fresh mint or a slice of lemon. Add sweetener if needed.

PUMPKIN SPICE COFFEE

Who needs those sugary, take-out lattes? High in healthy fats, this creamy, spiced coffee is a full meal in a mug.

1 SERVING	5 MINS	5 MINS

Prepare the coffee. Add it to a blender with the remaining ingredients. Pulse until smooth and frothy. Add sweeteners or top with whipped cream or coconut milk, if you wish.

INGREDIENTS

½ cup (120 ml/4.1 fl oz) black coffee

1 tablespoon (20 g/0.7 oz) pumpkin puree

¼ cup (60 ml/2 fl oz) heavy whipping cream or coconut milk

1 tablespoon (15 ml/0.5 fl oz) MCT oil or coconut oil

½ teaspoon unsweetened vanilla extract

1 teaspoon pumpkin spice mix (ground cinnamon, nutmeg, cloves, ginger, allspice)

3 to 5 drops liquid stevia or 1 tablespoon (10 g/0.4 oz) erythritol or Swerve

Optional: whipped cream or coconut milk for topping

NUTRITION FACTS PER SERVING

Total carbs: 5 g

Fiber: 1.7 g

Net carbs: 3.3 g

Protein: 1.6 g

Fat: 36.1 g

Energy: 347 kcal

Macronutrient ratio: Calories from carbs (4%), protein (2%), fat (94%)

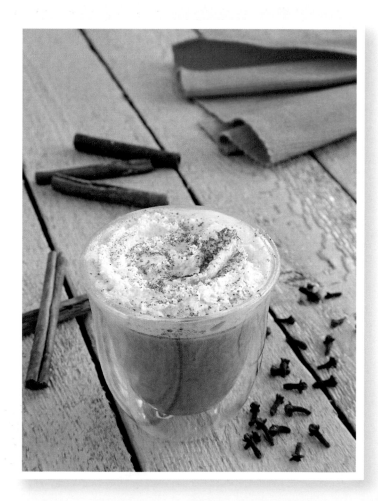

CHAI TEA TURMERIC LATTE

This rich chai tea latte is laden with turmeric, which is prized for its anti-inflammatory properties and which may promote stomach, liver, and skin health.

1 SERVING	10 MINS	10 MINS

INGREDIENTS

½ teaspoon ground ginger (or 1 teaspoon fresh)

¼ teaspoon cinnamon

2 cardamom pods

1 vanilla bean or 1 teaspoon powdered vanilla extract

Pinch each of freshly ground black pepper and salt

1½ cups (360 ml/12.2 fl oz) water

¼ cup (60 ml/2 fl oz) coconut milk or heavy whipping cream

1 teaspoon ground turmeric

1 tablespoon (15 ml/0.5 fl oz) MCT oil or coconut oil

Optional: 3 to 5 drops liquid stevia or 1 tablespoon (10 g/ 0.4 oz) erythritol or Swerve

Optional: whipped cream or coconut milk with cinnamon on top

First, prepare the chai tea concentrate. Place the ginger, cinnamon, cardamom, vanilla extract (or seeds scraped from the vanilla bean), black pepper, and salt into a saucepan. Add the water and bring to a boil. Reduce the heat and boil until it reduces by about half. When done, remove the pan from the heat and pour the liquid through a fine-mesh sieve. Discard the spices.

Prepare the turmeric milk. Mix the coconut milk with the ground turmeric in saucepan and bring to a boil. Simmer on low heat for about 5 minutes.

Pour the chai tea concentrate, turmeric milk, MCT oil, and liquid stevia, if using, into a blender and pulse until frothy—blending will prevent the oil from floating on top. Transfer to a glass and enjoy hot. Top with whipped cream or coconut milk, if you like.

NUTRITION FACTS PER SERVING

Total carbs: 3.9 g   **Protein:** 1.4 g

Fiber: 0.7 g   **Fat:** 25.3 g

Net carbs: 3.2 g   **Energy:** 237 kcal

Macronutrient ratio: Calories from carbs (5%), protein (2%), fat (93%)

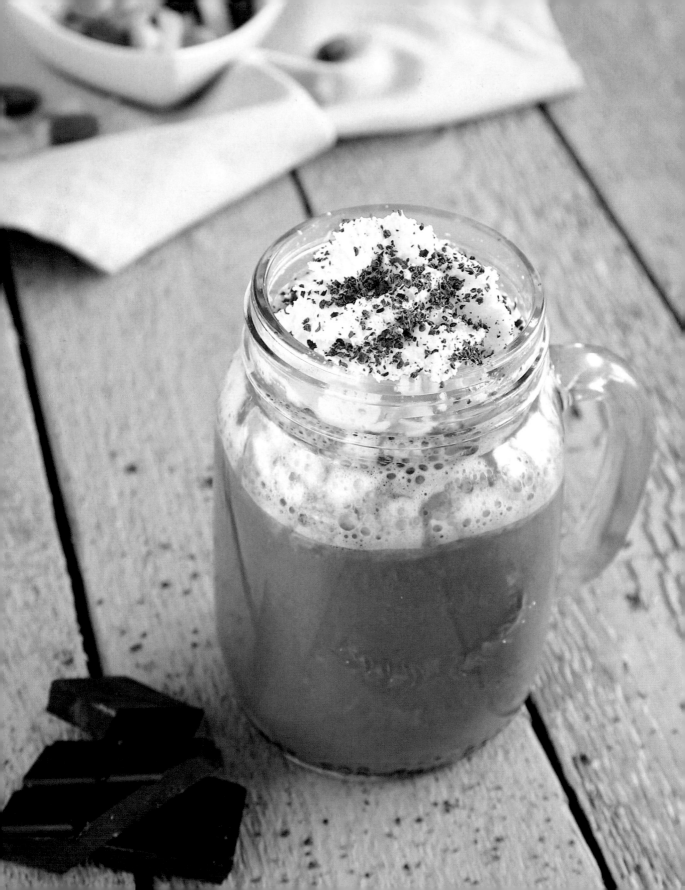

CREAMY HOT CHOCOLATE

Treat yourself to this low-carb hot chocolate on a cold winter's night or try it for breakfast: it's substantial enough to stand in for a full meal.

1 SERVING	5 MINS	5 MINS

INGREDIENTS

¼ cup (60 ml/2 fl oz) coconut milk or heavy whipping cream

¾ cup (180 ml/6.1 fl oz) water or almond milk

2 tablespoons (30 g/1.1 oz) Toasted Nut Butter (page 39) or Chocolate Hazelnut Butter (page 43)

2 tablespoons (10 g/0.4 oz) unsweetened cacao powder

Pinch cayenne pepper

1 tablespoon (15 ml/0.5 fl oz) MCT oil or coconut oil

Optional: 3 to 5 drops liquid stevia or 1 tablespoon (10 g/0.4 oz) erythritol or Swerve

Optional: whipped cream or coconut milk and grated dark chocolate on top

Pour the coconut milk and water into a saucepan and bring to a boil over medium heat. Add the nut butter, cacao powder, and cayenne pepper and mix well. Remove from the heat and add the MCT oil. Mix until well combined and pour into a cup or a serving glass. If you like, add the optional sweetener and then top with whipped cream or coconut milk and a dash of grated dark chocolate.

NUTRITION FACTS PER SERVING

Total carbs: 13.4 g   **Protein:** 7.1 g

Fiber: 7 g   **Fat:** 46.7 g

Net carbs: 6.4 g   **Energy:** 453 kcal

Macronutrient ratio: Calories from carbs (5%), protein (6%), fat (89%)

EGGNOG

This traditional egg yolk-based drink is a perfect low-carb treat. Don't wait for the holiday season to give it a try!

	2 SERVINGS		**5 MINS**		**5 MINS**

INGREDIENTS

2 large egg yolks

10 to 15 drops liquid stevia or 2 tablespoons (20 g/0.7 oz) erythritol or Swerve, powdered

1 cup (240 ml/8.1 fl oz) heavy whipping cream or coconut milk

1 cup (240 ml/8.1 fl oz) almond milk

¼ cup (60 ml/2 fl oz) dark rum or brandy or 1 teaspoon rum extract

1 vanilla bean or 1 teaspoon vanilla extract

½ teaspoon nutmeg

¼ teaspoon cinnamon

Optional: 2 whipped egg whites plus ¼ cup (56 g/2 oz) whipped cream on top

NUTRITION FACTS PER SERVING

Total carbs: 6.2 g

Fiber: 1.6 g

Net carbs: 4.6 g

Protein: 5.6 g

Fat: 51.8 g

Energy: 581 kcal

Macronutrient ratio:
Calories from carbs (4%), protein (4%), fat (92%)

Here are four different ways to make Eggnog:

Classic: Whisk the egg yolk with the liquid stevia or erythritol until creamy. Add the cream, almond milk, and rum and stir well. Add the nutmeg, cinnamon, and vanilla. Serve chilled or with ice.

Alcohol-free eggnog: Follow the same recipe but use rum extract and add more water, almond milk, and cream, if needed.

Add egg whites: To use the egg whites, whisk them until they create soft peaks. Add more sweetener if needed. Serve on top of the eggnog or mix into it to create a fluffy texture.

Use cooked eggs: In a heat-resistant bowl, mix the egg yolks, half of the almond milk, and half of the cream. Add vanilla, nutmeg, cinnamon, and the sweetener. Put the bowl over a pot with boiling water and cook for 5 to 8 minutes, stirring constantly. Remove from heat and mix in the remaining cream and almond milk. Add the rum. Serve hot or refrigerate and serve with ice.

TIPS

- If you're using raw eggs, due to the slight risk of salmonella or other foodborne illness, you should use only fresh, properly refrigerated, clean, grade A or AA eggs with intact shells and avoid contact between the yolks or whites and the outside of the shell.
- You can make raw eggs safe by using pasteurized eggs. To pasteurize eggs at home, simply pour enough water in a saucepan to cover the eggs. Heat to about 140°F (60°C). Using a spoon, slowly place the eggs into the saucepan. Keep the eggs in the water for about 3 minutes. This should be enough to pasteurize the eggs and kill any potential bacteria. Let the eggs cool down and store in the fridge for 6 to 8 weeks.

BLACKBERRY COCONUT BARK

High in healthy fats, this Blackberry Coconut Bark is the perfect alternative to chocolate—and it makes a great low-carb pre-workout snack, too.

12 SERVINGS	10 MINS	10 MINS + CHILLING

INGREDIENTS

½ cup (30 g/1.1 oz) desiccated coconut, flaked

1 cup (250 g/8.8 oz) coconut butter

¼ cup (55 ml/1.9 fl oz) extra virgin coconut oil

¼ cup (60 g/2.1 oz) butter or more coconut oil

½ cup (70 g/2.5 oz) blackberries, unsweetened and frozen

¼ teaspoon salt

Optional: 2 tablespoons (20 g/ 0.7 oz) erythritol or Swerve and 15 to 20 drops liquid stevia

NUTRITION FACTS PER PIECE

Total carbs: 5.5 g

Fiber: 3.8 g

Net carbs: 1.7 g

Protein: 1.5 g

Fat: 21.7 g

Energy: 211 kcal

Macronutrient ratio: Calories from carbs (3%), protein (3%), fat (94%)

Toast the flaked coconut until golden in a pan over medium-high heat. Stir frequently to prevent burning. When done, set it aside.

Place the coconut butter, coconut oil, butter (or more coconut oil), powdered erythritol, and liquid stevia, if using, in a bowl and melt in a water bath. Make sure you use coconut butter (creamed coconut meat), not creamed coconut milk. To make the water bath, simply place the bowl over a pot with boiling water and stir until everything melts completely. The bowl has to be bigger than the saucepan, and the boiling water should not reach the bottom of the bowl; only the steam should heat the bowl.

Set a baking sheet over a medium plate. Pour the coconut mixture on the sheet and top with toasted coconut and frozen blackberries and season with salt. You can use fine or larger grains of salt.

Place in the fridge for at least 30 minutes or until set. When done, cut into 12 pieces and keep refrigerated for up to three days or freeze for up to three months.

TIP

Use raspberries, strawberries, or blueberries in place of the blackberries.

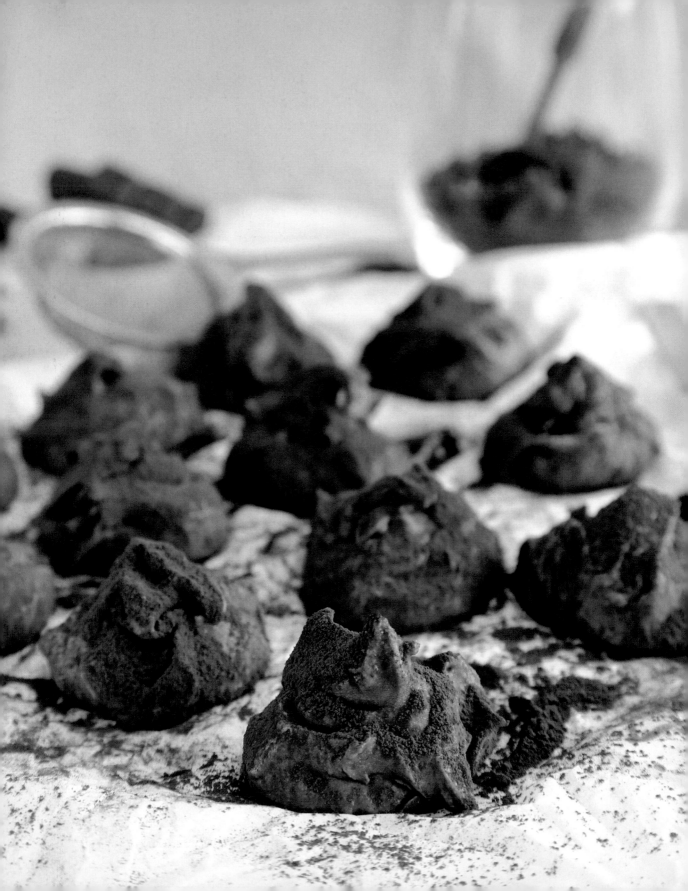

CHOCOLATE FAT BOMBS

Fat bombs are keto-friendly snacks: reach for a couple if you find it hard to boost your fat intake, or if you're on a fat fast.

15 TRUFFLES	10 MINS	10 MINS + CHILLING

INGREDIENTS

½ cup (125 g/4.4 oz) coconut butter

¼ cup (55 ml/1.9 fl oz) extra virgin coconut oil

½ cup (110 g/3.9 oz) butter or more coconut oil

3 tablespoons (25 g/0.9 oz) unsweetened cacao powder

15 to 20 drops liquid stevia

Optional: 2 tablespoons (20 g/0.7 oz) erythritol or Swerve, powdered

Optional: 1 teaspoon hazelnut, cherry, or almond extract, or pinch of cayenne pepper

NUTRITION FACTS PER TRUFFLE

Total carbs: 2.7 g

Fiber: 1.8 g

Net carbs: 1 g

Protein: 0.9 g

Fat: 14.4

Energy: 134 kcal

Macronutrient ratio: Calories from carbs (3%), protein (2%), fat (95%)

Let the coconut butter, coconut oil, and butter sit at room temperature to soften (but do not let melt). Make sure you use coconut butter for this recipe: that's creamed coconut meat, not creamed coconut milk.

Combine all the ingredients in a food processor, but keep some cacao aside for coating. Process until smooth.

Line a baking sheet with parchment paper (or any nonstick mat) and use a spoon to form 15 small truffles. Place in the fridge for 30 to 60 minutes.

Remove from the fridge and sift the remaining cacao powder over the fat bombs. Store in the fridge for up to a week or freeze for up to three months.

KETO CRÈME BRÛLÉE

My low-carb, paleo-friendly version of this popular dessert includes an extra ingredient that gives it a caramelized crust—just like the real thing!

 4 SERVINGS | **15 MINS** | **10 MINS** + CHILLING

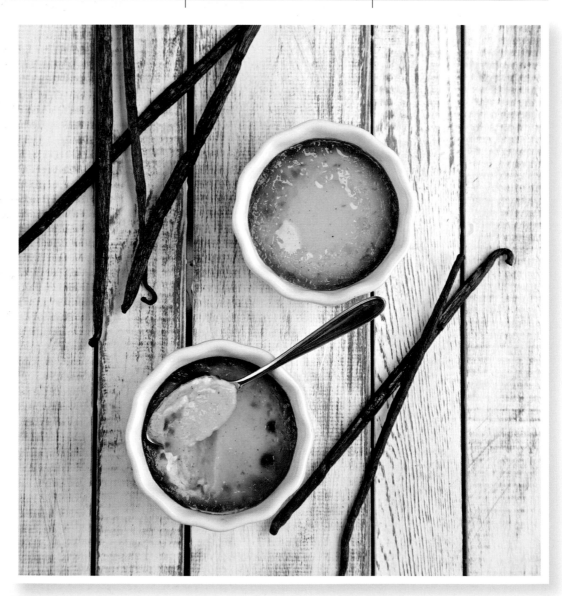

INGREDIENTS

Custard

2 cups (480 ml/16.2 fl oz) heavy whipping cream or coconut milk

2 vanilla beans or 2 teaspoons sugar-free vanilla extract

5 large egg yolks

¼ cup (40 g/1.4 oz) erythritol or Swerve

15 to 20 drops liquid stevia

Topping

6 teaspoons (20 g/0.7 oz) erythritol or Swerve

NUTRITION FACTS PER SERVING

Total carbs: 5.6 g

Fiber: 0.7 g

Net carbs: 4.8 g

Protein: 5.7 g

Fat: 51.2 g

Energy: 513 kcal

Macronutrient ratio:
Calories from carbs (4%), protein (5%), fat (91%)

Preheat the oven to 325°F (160°C, or gas mark 3). Pour the cream into a pan over medium heat.

Cut the vanilla beans lengthwise and unfold them (or add the sugar-free vanilla extract). Mix in the vanilla beans and simmer the cream for about 5 minutes. Lower the heat, if needed, to prevent the cream from boiling over. Take off the heat and set it aside.

Separate the egg yolks from the egg whites and reserve the egg whites for another use. Whisk the egg yolks together with the erythritol and liquid stevia. Keep some erythritol aside for the topping (1½ teaspoons per serving).

Slowly pour the hot cream into the egg yolks while whisking. Do not pour all of it in at once, or you'll risk cooking the egg. Use a sieve to remove the tiny vanilla seeds; discard them.

Place four ramekins in a deep casserole dish filled with 1 to 2 cups (235 to 475 ml/8 to 16 fl oz) of hot water, enough to cover the cups up to about a third. Fill the ramekins about three-quarters full with the mixture. Cover the casserole dish with parchment paper. Make sure there is a small gap—do not cover too tightly.

Cook in the oven for 40 to 45 minutes. When done, the custard should be set on the outside and soft in the middle. Remove from the oven. Take the ramekins out of the water and place on a cooling rack until they reach room temperature. Place in the fridge until chilled.

Take the ramekins out of the fridge 30 minutes before you are ready to serve and spread 1½ teaspoons of erythritol on top of each. Place under a broiler set to high for about 3 to 5 minutes to caramelize, or use a blow torch.

QUICK RASPBERRY ICE CREAM

*A healthy summer refresher, this berry-laden
ice cream doesn't require an ice-cream maker,
and it takes less than 5 minutes to make.*

 1 SERVINGS | 5 MINS | 5 MINS

INGREDIENTS

½ cup (75 g/2.6 oz)
raspberries, unsweetened and
frozen

¼ cup (25 g/0.9 oz) whey
protein or egg white protein
powder: berry, vanilla or
unflavored

¼ cup (60 ml/2 fl oz) coconut
milk or heavy whipping cream

1 tablespoon (15 ml/0.5 fl oz)
MCT oil

Optional: 5 to 10 drops
liquid stevia

NUTRITION FACTS PER SERVING

Total carbs: 7.7 g

Fiber: 1.9 g

Net carbs: 5.8 g

Protein: 21.9 g

Fat: 25.3 g

Energy: 330 kcal

Macronutrient ratio:
Calories from carbs (7%),
protein (26%), fat (67%)

Place all the ingredients into a blender and pulse until smooth.
When done, eat immediately or place the ice cream in an airtight
container and store in the freezer.

TIP

Try using other berries: strawberries, blackberries, and raspberries are
the lowest in net carbs. You may not need to use any sweetener, as the
berries should be enough to give the ice cream a naturally sweet taste.

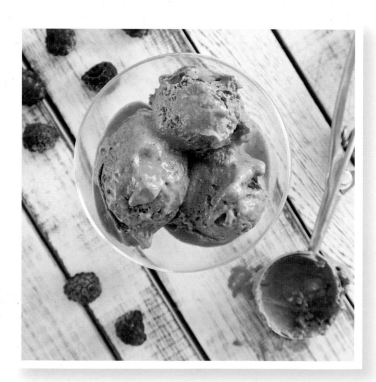

BLACKBERRY & RHUBARB CRISP

Blackberries and rhubarb are some of the best low-carb fruits. Combine them in this grain-free crisp, and serve with a dollop of full-fat yogurt or sour cream.

12 SERVINGS	20 MINS	1 HOUR

INGREDIENTS

2 cups (300 g/10.6 oz) each rhubarb, and blackberries, fresh or frozen

¼ cup (40 g/1.4 oz) erythritol or Swerve

15 to 20 drops liquid stevia

½ teaspoon each cinnamon and ground ginger

2 tablespoons (16 g/0.6 oz) ground chia seeds

Crisp

1½ cups (150 g/5.3 oz) almond flour

5.3 ounces (150 g) macadamia nuts, roughly chopped

½ cup (50 g/1.8 oz) pecans or walnuts, roughly chopped

¼ cup (25 g/0.9 oz) whey protein or egg white protein powder, vanilla or unflavored

½ teaspoon cinnamon

¼ teaspoon salt

⅓ cup (50 g/1.8 oz) erythritol or Swerve

1 large egg white

¼ cup (56 g/2 oz) butter or coconut oil, chilled

10 to 15 drops liquid stevia

Preheat the oven to 400°F (200°C, or gas mark 6). Wash and slice the rhubarb. Wash the blackberries if using fresh. Place the blackberries and rhubarb into a casserole dish. Sprinkle evenly with erythritol, liquid stevia, cinnamon, and ginger and mix well. Place in the oven and bake for about 20 minutes. Mix once or twice to prevent burning. When done, set it aside.

Reduce the oven temperature to 300°F (150°C, or gas mark 2). Add the ground chia seeds to the baked fruit and mix well.

Meanwhile, prepare the crisp. Roughly chop the nuts. Mix the almond flour, chopped macadamia nuts, walnuts or pecans, whey protein, cinnamon, salt, and erythritol and mix well. Add the egg white, chilled butter, and liquid stevia.

Using your hands, mix well until you create a crumbly dough. Sprinkle pieces of the dough over the baked fruit and return to the oven. Bake for 20 minutes or until the crisp is golden. Keep an eye on it—nuts burn easily. Let it stand a few minutes and then serve.

NUTRITION FACTS PER SERVING

Total carbs: 9.7 g **Protein:** 7.1 g **Macronutrient ratio:** Calories from carbs (7%), protein (11%), fat (82%)

Fiber: 5.4 g **Fat:** 22.2 g

Net carbs: 4.3 g **Energy:** 248 kcal

STRAWBERRY CHEESE BREAD

This recipe was inspired by my Pumpkin & Orange Cheese Bread, one of the most popular recipes on my blog.

10 SLICES	15 MINS	50 MINS + CHILLING

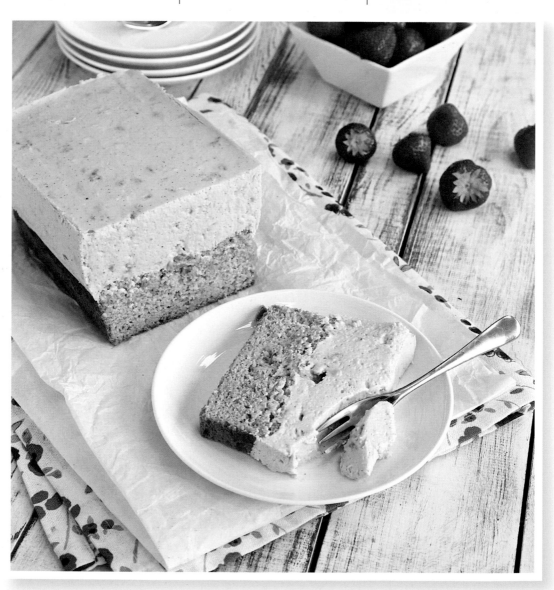

INGREDIENTS

Bread Layer

3 large eggs, separated

⅓ cup (50 g/1.8 oz) erythritol or Swerve

15 to 20 drops liquid stevia

1 vanilla bean or 1 teaspoon unsweetened vanilla extract

3 tablespoons (45 g/1.6 oz) butter, ghee or coconut oil, softened

¾ cup (75 g/2.6 oz) almond flour

¼ cup (30 g/1.1 oz) coconut flour

½ teaspoon baking soda

¼ cup (60 ml/2 fl oz) coconut milk or almond milk

1 teaspoon cream of tartar

Cheese Layer

1½ cups (225 g/7.9 oz) strawberries, fresh or frozen

17.6 ounces (500 g) cream cheese

¼ cup (60 g/2.1 oz) sour cream

1 tablespoon (15 ml/0.5 fl oz) lemon juice

1 vanilla bean or 1 teaspoon unsweetened vanilla extract

⅓ cup (50 g/1.8 oz) erythritol

15 to 20 drops liquid stevia

¼ cup (60 ml/2 fl oz) hot water

2 tablespoons (14 g/0.5 oz) gelatin or 2 teaspoons agar powder

Preheat the oven to 350°F (175°C, or gas mark 4). Line a loaf pan with parchment paper or use a silicone loaf pan. First, prepare the bread layer. Separate the egg whites from the egg yolks. In the bowl with the egg yolks, add the powdered erythritol and liquid stevia. Cut the vanilla bean lengthwise and scrape the seeds into the bowl with the yolks. Mix until creamy. Add the softened butter and stir until well combined.

Add the almond flour, coconut flour, and baking soda and combine well. Sift the dry ingredients, if needed, to avoid any lumps in the dough.

In a separate bowl, whisk the egg whites with the cream of tartar until they create soft peaks. Add to the dough and gently fold in. Be careful not to deflate the egg whites.

Pour the dough into the loaf pan and transfer to the oven. Bake for about 30 minutes until the bread layer is firm and the top is golden. When done, remove from the oven and let cool on a rack before adding the cheese layer.

To prepare the cheese layer, wash the strawberries and puree. Pour them into a bowl together with the cream cheese and sour cream. Add the lemon juice, vanilla extract, erythritol, and liquid stevia.

In a small bowl, combine the hot water and gelatin. Let it dissolve and then slowly drizzle in the cream cheese mixture while beating. Using a food processor, mix on high speed to prevent the gelatin from clumping.

If you're using agar powder, dissolve ½ tablespoon (5 g/0.2 oz) of agar powder (not whole agar flakes) in ¼ cup (60 ml/2 fl oz) of hot water and bring to a boil. Simmer for 1 to 2 minutes and then drizzle into the cheese layer ingredients while beating with a mixer set to high speed.

Pour the cheese mixture over the chilled bread layer and let set in the fridge for at least 4 hours or overnight before slicing and serving.

NUTRITION FACTS PER SLICE

Total carbs: 7.4 g
Fiber: 2.4 g
Net carbs: 5 g

Protein: 9.1 g
Fat: 25.7 g
Energy: 268 kcal

Macronutrient ratio: Calories from carbs (7%), protein (13%), fat (80%)

CHOCOLATE CREPES
WITH CHANTILLY CREAM

These glorious chocolate crepes with Chantilly cream, chocolate sauce, and toasted almonds make a truly special dessert—perfect for birthdays and other special occasions.

6 SERVINGS	15 MINS	20 MINS

INGREDIENTS

Crepes
¼ cup (25 g/0.9 oz) unsweetened cacao powder

¼ cup (25 g/0.9 oz) whey protein or egg white protein powder

2 tablespoons (20 g/0.7 oz) erythritol or Swerve, powdered

Pinch salt

1 vanilla bean or 1 teaspoon unsweetened vanilla extract

4 large eggs

3 tablespoons (45 g/1.6 oz) butter, ghee or coconut oil plus more for greasing

¼ cup (60 ml/2 fl oz) almond milk

10 to 15 drops liquid stevia

Chocolate Sauce
½ bar (50 g/1.8 oz) extra dark chocolate (85% cacao or more)

1 tablespoon (15 g/0.5 oz) coconut oil or butter

2 tablespoons (30 ml/1 fl oz) cream or coconut milk

½ cup (30 g/1.1 oz) flaked and toasted almonds

(continued)

Start with the crepes. Sift the cacao powder into a bowl and add the protein powder, powdered erythritol, and salt. Stir until well combined.

Cut the vanilla bean lengthwise and scrape the seeds into the powder mixture. Crack in the eggs and add two tablespoons (28 g/1 oz) of melted butter or coconut oil, almond milk, and liquid stevia. Whisk well until smooth and creamy. Leave to stand for about 10 minutes before making the crepes.

Meanwhile, prepare the chocolate sauce. Break the chocolate into small pieces and add to a heatproof bowl together with the coconut oil or butter. Place over a pan filled with simmering water: make sure the water doesn't touch the bowl. Slowly melt, stirring frequently. Remove from the heat and slowly pour in the cream or coconut milk and stir until well combined. Set aside and keep warm.

If not using already toasted sliced almonds, dry roast the almond slices for just 1 to 2 minutes until lightly browned and crispy.

Prepare the Chantilly cream by whipping the heavy whipping cream. Slowly sift in the powdered erythritol and add the liquid stevia and vanilla extract while whipping. Refrigerate.

Grease a medium nonstick pan with a small amount of coconut oil or ghee (do not use butter—it will burn). Stir the crepe mixture so it's well combined. When the pan is hot, pour in a small ladleful of the batter to create a crepe that's about 8 inches (20 cm) in diameter.

Chantilly Cream

1 cup (240 ml/8.1 fl oz) heavy whipping cream or creamed coconut milk

¼ cup (40 g/1.4 oz) erythritol or Swerve, powdered

10 to 15 drops liquid stevia

1 vanilla bean or 1 teaspoon unsweetened vanilla extract

NUTRITION FACTS PER SERVING

Total carbs: 8.5 g

Fiber: 3.3 g

Net carbs: 5.2 g

Protein: 11.4 g

Fat: 36.7 g

Energy: 395 kcal

Macronutrient ratio:
Calories from carbs (5%), protein (12%), fat (83%)

Swirl the pan or use the ladle to spread the batter into a thin layer. Cook for about a minute or until the batter is set. Flip over using a spatula. Cook for another 30 seconds. Transfer to a plate and cover with a towel to keep warm. Repeat for the remaining five crepes and grease the pan again if needed.

To serve, spread the whipped cream over half of each crepe. Fold each half of the crepes over the cream and then fold again in quarters. Drizzle with the chocolate sauce and sprinkle with the toasted almonds.

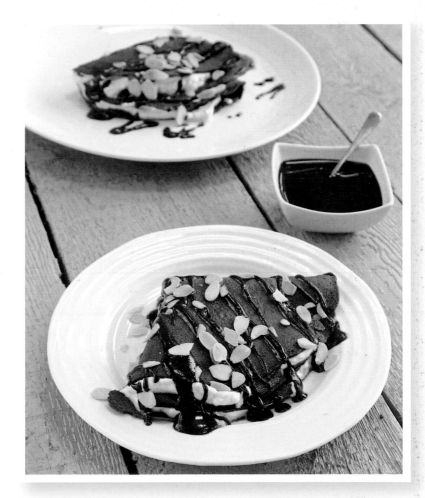

FUDGY GRASSHOPPER BROWNIES

These decadent, mint-chocolate brownies are the answer to your sugar cravings: a single piece will fill you up for hours!

 16 SERVINGS | **20 MINS** | **45 MINS** + CHILLING

INGREDIENTS

Brownie layer

1 bar (100 g/3.5 oz) extra dark chocolate (85% cacao or more)

4.4 ounces (125 g) butter, ghee or coconut oil

3 large eggs

15 to 20 drops liquid stevia

¾ cup (120 g/4.2 oz) erythritol or Swerve, powdered

1 cup (100 g/3.5 oz) almond flour

½ cup plus 1 tablespoon (45 g/1.6 oz) unsweetened cacao powder

¼ cup (30 g/1.1 oz) ground chia seeds

½ teaspoon baking soda

1 teaspoon cream of tartar

Mint Layer

7.1 ounces (200 g) coconut butter, softened

1 cup (75 g/2.6 oz) dried shredded coconut

¼ cup (40 g/1.4 oz) erythritol or Swerve, powdered

¼ cup (60 ml/2 fl oz) coconut milk or heavy whipping cream

10 to 15 drops liquid stevia

¼ cup (24 g/0.9 oz) fresh mint or more to taste

1 teaspoon to 1 tablespoon sugar-free mint extract (to taste)

(continued)

First, prepare the brownie base. Preheat the oven to 350°F (175°C, or gas mark 4). Break the chocolate into small pieces and add to a heatproof bowl with the butter. Place over a pan filled with simmering water and make sure the water doesn't touch the bowl: only the steam should heat the bowl. Slowly melt while stirring. When most of the chocolate is melted, remove the pan from the burner and let the mixture continue to melt while stirring. The chocolate mixture should not be hot when added to the dough.

Place the eggs, liquid stevia, and powdered erythritol into a bowl and whisk until well combined. Beat in the chocolate mixture and gently fold in the almond flour, cacao powder, ground chia seeds, baking soda, and cream of tartar and process well.

Pour into an 8 × 8 inch pan (20 × 20 cm) lined with parchment paper or use a silicone pan. Bake for 20 to 25 minutes. When done, remove from the oven and set on a cooling rack.

While the brownie base is cooling, prepare the mint layer. Place the softened coconut butter, shredded coconut, powdered erythritol, coconut milk, liquid stevia, mint and mint extract into a blender and pulse until smooth. If you prefer more texture, leave some shredded coconut aside and stir into the mixture after blending. The amount of mint depends on your palate and will not affect the amount of carbs per serving. Once the brownie layer has cooled, keep it in the baking pan and spread the mint layer over it.

Now, prepare the chocolate crust. Break the chocolate into small pieces and place in a bowl with the coconut oil. Pour the coconut milk or cream into a small saucepan and bring to a simmer over medium heat. Once simmering, pour the milk over the chocolate and coconut oil and mix until smooth and creamy. Set aside to cool and thicken slightly. When cool, spread on top of the mint layer, then refrigerate the brownies for 1 to 2 hours or until set before slicing.

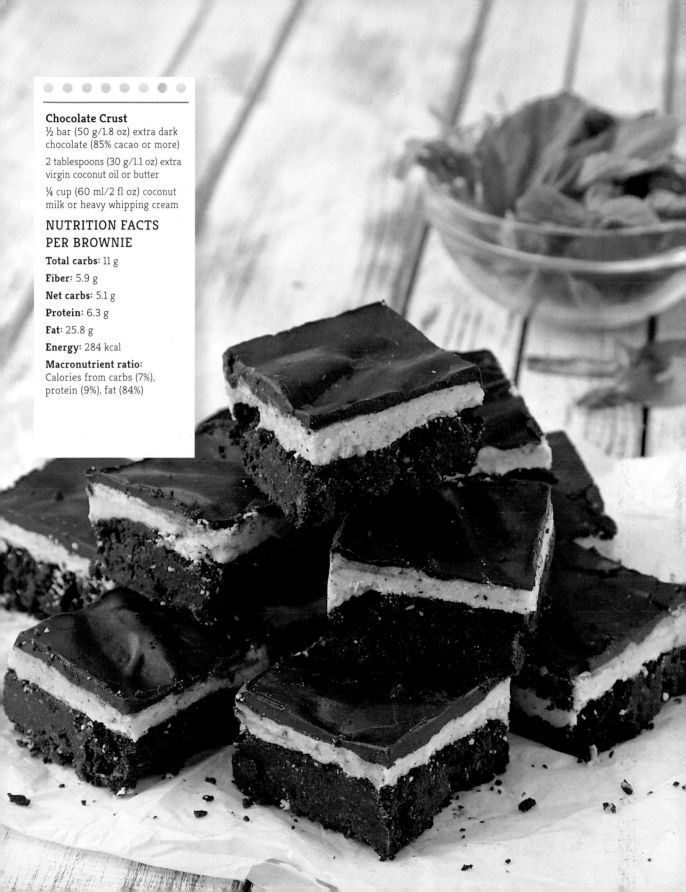

Chocolate Crust

½ bar (50 g/1.8 oz) extra dark chocolate (85% cacao or more)

2 tablespoons (30 g/1.1 oz) extra virgin coconut oil or butter

¼ cup (60 ml/2 fl oz) coconut milk or heavy whipping cream

NUTRITION FACTS PER BROWNIE

Total carbs: 11 g

Fiber: 5.9 g

Net carbs: 5.1 g

Protein: 6.3 g

Fat: 25.8 g

Energy: 284 kcal

Macronutrient ratio: Calories from carbs (7%), protein (9%), fat (84%)

CHOCOLATE CHIP & ORANGE COOKIES

*Chocolate and citrus is an underused combination,
and it's lovely in these easy-to-make, grain-free cookies.*

12 COOKIES	10 MINS	25 MINS

INGREDIENTS

1 cup (100 g/3.5 oz) almond flour

½ recipe (about ¾ cup/ 200 g/7.1 oz) Toasted Nut Butter (page 39)

¼ cup (40 g/1.4 oz) erythritol or Swerve

15 to 20 drops liquid stevia

2 tablespoons (12 g/0.4 oz) orange peel (or 1 tablespoon dried)

1 tablespoon (8 g/0.3 oz) ginger

1 large egg

½ teaspoon cinnamon

½ teaspoon baking soda

1 teaspoon cream of tartar

¼ teaspoon salt

⅓ cup (60 g/2.1 oz) extra dark chocolate chips (85% cacao or more)

Preheat the oven to 350°F (175°C, or gas mark 4). Place all the ingredients except for the chocolate chips in a bowl and mix until well combined. Add the chocolate chips to the bowl and mix until well incorporated.

Form 12 equal balls and place them on a baking sheet lined with parchment paper. Using your hand or a spatula, flatten each of the balls to create a cookie. If any chocolate chips fall out, press them back into the top of the cookies.

Bake for 12 to 15 minutes or until the tops are golden. When done, remove from the oven and set aside to cool.

TIP

Shape the dough into a roughly 2-inch-thick (5 cm) roll, cut into ½-inch (1.3 cm) slices, wrap in parchment paper, twist the ends, and store in the fridge for up to three days or in the freezer for longer. Anytime you want to make fresh cookies, simply set the frozen dough on a baking sheet lined with parchment paper and bake 12 to 15 minutes for refrigerated dough or 15 to 18 minutes for frozen dough.

NUTRITION FACTS PER COOKIE

Total carbs: 6.9 g   **Protein:** 5 g   **Macronutrient ratio:**
Fiber: 3.5 g   **Fat:** 17.6 g   Calories from carbs (7%), protein (10%),
Net carbs: 3.4 g   **Energy:** 191 kcal   fat (83%)

DOUBLE CHOCOLATE MUFFINS

A muffin recipe that calls for avocado. Really? It's not as odd as it sounds! Packed with healthy fats, avocado makes these chocolatey muffins so rich and moist.

8 MUFFINS	10 MINS	30 TO 35 MINS

INGREDIENTS

Dry Ingredients

⅓ cup (40 g/1.4 oz) coconut flour

1 cup (100 g/3.5 oz) almond flour

⅓ cup (30 g/1.1 oz) unsweetened cacao powder

½ cup (80 g/2.8 oz) erythritol or Swerve

1 teaspoon each cinnamon and baking soda

2 teaspoons cream of tartar

⅓ cup (60 g/2.1 oz) dark chocolate (85% cacao or more), roughly chopped

Wet Ingredients

2 medium (250 g/8.8 oz) avocados

15 to 20 drops stevia

4 large eggs

2 tablespoons (30 ml/1 fl oz) coconut milk or heavy whipping cream

Preheat the oven to 350°F (175°C, or gas mark 4). Halve, deseed, and peel the avocados and place them into a food processor. Pulse until smooth and creamy.

Sift together the coconut flour, almond flour, and cacao powder. Add the erythritol, cinnamon, baking soda, and cream of tartar and mix well.

Add the liquid stevia, eggs, coconut milk, and pureed avocado and process until well combined. Finally, roughly chop the chocolate and add to the mixture. Reserve a few pieces for topping.

Scoop the muffin batter into a silicon muffin pan or a regular muffin pan lined with paper cups greased with a small amount of coconut oil or ghee.

Top with the reserved chocolate pieces and place in the oven. Bake for about 25 minutes or until the tops are crispy and the muffins are firm.

Remove from the oven and let the muffins cool on a rack before serving. Keep at room temperature covered with a kitchen towel for up to three days or place in an airtight container and refrigerate for longer.

NUTRITION FACTS PER MUFFIN

Total carbs: 12.2 g   **Protein:** 9 g   **Macronutrient ratio:**
Fiber: 6.6 g   **Fat:** 19 g   Calories from carbs (10%), protein (16%), fat (74%)
Net carbs: 5.7 g   **Energy:** 237 kcal

BOSTON CREAM PIE

My Boston Cream Pie does require a bit of work, but it's so worth it. With custard filling sandwiched between sponge cake halves and coated in dark chocolate ganache, this one's sure to satisfy even the most stubborn sweet tooth.

12 SERVINGS	35 MINS	2 HOURS

INGREDIENTS

Sponge base

¼ cup (30 g/1.1 oz) coconut flour

2 cups (200 g/7.1 oz) almond flour

¼ cup (25 g/0.9 oz) whey protein or egg white protein: vanilla or unflavored

1 teaspoon baking soda

2 teaspoons cream of tartar

¼ teaspoon salt

½ cup (80 g/2.8 oz) erythritol or Swerve

¼ cup (56 g/2 oz) butter or coconut oil, softened

4 large eggs

1 vanilla bean or 1 teaspoon unsweetened vanilla extract

½ cup (120 ml/4.1 fl oz) almond milk

15 to 20 drops liquid stevia

¼ cup (56 g/2 oz) butter or coconut oil

(continued)

Preheat the oven to 350°F (175°C, or gas mark 4). Line a cake pan with a removable bottom with parchment paper.

Sift the dry ingredients for the sponge base into a bowl and mix until well combined.

Beat together the erythritol and softened butter or coconut oil. Gradually add the eggs and beat until light and creamy. Cut the vanilla bean lengthwise and scrape the seeds into the mixture. Slowly pour in the almond milk, and while whisking, add the liquid stevia, then fold in the dry ingredients.

Pour the batter into the cake pan and transfer to the oven. Bake for 30 to 35 minutes or until the top is golden brown and the inside is fluffy and firm.

Meanwhile, prepare the custard cream filling. Pour the cream and ¼ cup (60 ml/2 fl oz) of almond milk into a saucepan and gently bring to a boil over a medium heat. Mix the remaining almond milk with the arrowroot powder and set aside.

In a separate bowl, beat together the egg yolks, powdered erythritol, liquid stevia, vanilla extract, and salt. Pour two ladlefuls, one at a time, of the hot cream into the beaten eggs, stirring constantlty. Then, pour the egg mixture into the remaining hot cream and keep stirring to prevent the eggs from scrambling.

Vanilla Cream Custard

1 cup (240 ml/8.1 fl oz) heavy whipping cream or coconut milk

½ cup (120 ml/4.1 fl oz) almond milk

1 tablespoon (9 g/0.3 oz) arrowroot powder

4 large egg yolks

¼ cup (40 g/1.4 oz) erythritol or Swerve, powdered

10 to 15 drops liquid stevia

1 vanilla bean or 1 teaspoon unsweetened vanilla extract

Pinch salt

Chocolate Ganaches

1 bar (100 g/3.5 oz) extra dark chocolate (85% cacao or more)

2 tablespoons (30 g/1.1 oz) butter or coconut oil

1 vanilla bean or 1 teaspoon unsweetened vanilla extract

¼ cup (60 ml/2 fl oz) heavy whipping cream or coconut milk

NUTRITION FACTS PER SLICE

Total carbs: 9 g

Fiber: 3.2 g

Net carbs: 5.8 g

Protein: 10.2 g

Fat: 35.4 g

Energy: 386 kcal

Macronutrient ratio: Calories from carbs (6%), protein (11%), fat (83%)

Cook and stir constantly until the filling starts to thicken. Then, add the arrowroot mixed with almond milk—you may need to stir it again before pouring it in the custard. Cook for another minute and remove from the heat. Add the butter or coconut oil and mix until well combined. Cover the surface with plastic wrap, let it cool, and then refrigerate. Alternatively, place the bowl in ice water and stir until chilled.

When the cake is ready to be assembled, make the chocolate ganache. Break the chocolate into small pieces and place in a bowl with the butter or coconut oil and vanilla extract. Heat the cream over a medium heat and, when boiling, pour over the chocolate and butter. Mix until smooth and creamy. Leave to cool down slightly before spreading on the cake.

Cut the cake horizontally through the middle and spread the vanilla custard cream filling over the bottom half. Place the other half on top and pour the ganache over it, allowing it to drip down the sides. Leave to set or refrigerate before cutting into slices.

TIPS

- You can substitute coconut oil for butter or ghee in most recipes. However, when cool, coconut oil tends to be harder than butter: keep this in mind when using it to make frostings, glazes, and ganaches.

- Don't waste the egg whites! You can use them to make Fluffy Grain-free Sunflower Bread (page 20), Ultimate Keto Bread (page 19), or Ultimate Keto Buns (page 26).

LEMON MERINGUE TARTLETS

You'll love the crispy almond crust, zesty lemon curd filling, and fluffy meringue in this grain- and sugar-free adaptation of the classic dessert.

8 TARTLETS	30 MINS	50 MINS + CHILLING

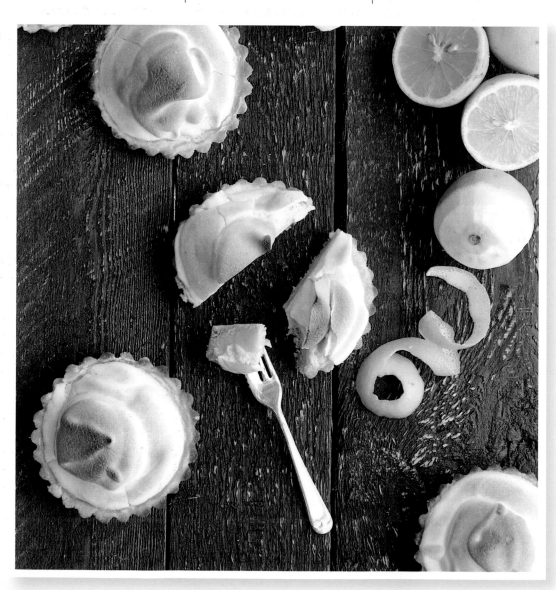

INGREDIENTS

Lemon Curd Filling

Zest from 3 lemons

Juice from 4 lemons (¾ cup [180 ml/6.1 fl oz] lemon juice)

6 large egg yolks

½ cup (80 g/2.8 oz) erythritol or Swerve, powdered

15 to 20 drops liquid stevia

1 tablespoon (9 g/0.3 oz) arrowroot powder or gelatin powder

2 tablespoons water

3½ ounces (100 g) butter or extra virgin coconut oil

Tartlet Base

1¾ cups (175 g/6.2 oz) almond flour

¼ cup (25 g/0.9 oz) whey protein or egg white protein powder

¼ cup (40 g/1.4 oz) erythritol or Swerve, powdered

1 large egg

2 tablespoons (30 g/1.1 oz) coconut oil or butter, melted

Pinch salt

Meringue

4 large egg whites

¼ teaspoon cream of tartar

⅓ cup (50 g/1.8 oz) erythritol or Swerve, powdered

NUTRITION FACTS PER TART

Total carbs: 9.2 g

Fiber: 2.9 g

Net carbs: 6.4 g

Protein: 12.4 g

Fat: 29.1 g

Energy: 332 kcal

Macronutrient ratio: Calories from carbs (7%), protein (15%), fat (78%)

First, prepare the lemon curd filling. Zest and juice the lemons and set aside. Place the egg yolks with the powdered erythritol and liquid stevia in a heat-resistant bowl and beat well. Place the bowl over a saucepan filled with simmering water and stir constantly; make sure the water doesn't touch the bottom of the bowl.

Add the fresh lemon juice and zest and keep stirring for 8 to 10 minutes until the curd starts to thicken. Mix the arrowroot with 2 tablespoons of water and pour into the lemon curd filling, stirring constantly. Cook for another minute or two and take off the heat. Add the butter and stir it in well. Cover with plastic wrap and refrigerate until thickened.

Preheat the oven to 350°F (175°C, or gas mark 4). Prepare the dough for the tartlet base. Place the almond flour, protein powder, powdered erythritol, coconut oil, egg, and salt into a bowl and process until well combined.

Separate the dough into eight equal pieces and press in the bottom of each 4 inch (10 cm) tartlet pan. (Use tartlet pans with removable bottoms or a silicone pan. Or, use a regular pan and make a large meringue pie.) If the dough is too sticky, wet your fingers to press it into the tart pan. Press toward the edges to create a bowl shape so that the tartlet can hold the lemon curd filling. You should be able to create a very thin, crispy pastry with the risen edges. Make sure there are no gaps in the batter so that the filling cannot leak through once poured in.

Bake the tartlets the oven for about 10 minutes. Watch them carefully, since almonds can burn easily. When done, remove from the oven and cool on a rack.

When the lemon curd is chilled and thick enough, preheat the oven to 325°F (160°C, or gas mark 3). Prepare the meringue topping. Beat the egg whites with the cream of tartar and gradually add the powdered erythritol until the egg whites create soft peaks. Do not overbeat; the meringue will be too stiff.

Fill each tartlet with about 2 tablespoons (28 g/1 oz) of the lemon curd filling and evenly distribute the rest. Top with the fluffy meringue. Bake for 15 to 20 minutes or until the meringues start to brown. You can use a blowtorch to finish browning the meringue tops. When done, carefully remove the tartlets from the oven and let cool. Store them in the fridge for up to five days.

TIRAMISU TRIFLE

This low-carb version of the famous Italian dessert looks beautiful when it's presented in single-serving parfaits.

6 SERVINGS	20 MINS	35 MINS + CHILLING

INGREDIENTS

Ladyfingers
3 large eggs, separated

2 tablespoons (20 g/0.7 oz) erythritol or Swerve, powdered

15 to 20 drops stevia

1 large egg white

¼ cup and 1 tablespoon (35 g/1.2 oz) coconut flour

⅓ cup (35 g/1.2 oz) almond flour

Mascarpone Layer
4 large eggs, separated

Pinch salt

½ cup (80 g/2.8 oz) erythritol or Swerve, powdered

10 to 15 drops stevia

1 cup (250 g/8.8 oz) mascarpone cheese or creamed coconut milk

6 teaspoons (10 g/0.4 oz) unsweetened cacao powder

Coffee Liquor
½ cup (120 ml/4.1 fl oz) freshly brewed strong black coffee

¼ cup (60 ml/2 fl oz) dark rum or brandy (or 1 tablespoon rum extract)

2 tablespoons (20 g/0.7 oz) erythritol or Swerve

10 to 15 drops stevia

Preheat the oven to 375°F (190°C, or gas mark 5). Start by making the ladyfingers. Line a 10 × 10 inch (25 × 25 cm) pan with parchment paper. Separate the egg whites from the egg yolks. Cream the yolks in a bowl with the powdered erythritol and liquid stevia until pale and creamy.

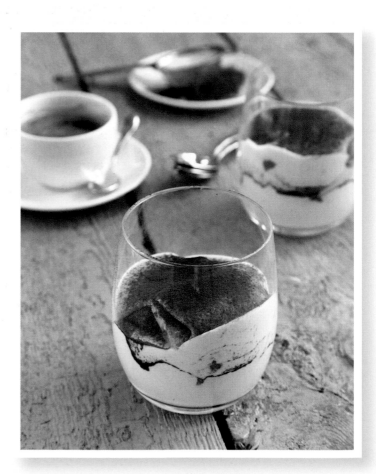

In a separate bowl, whisk the four egg whites until they create soft peaks. Gently fold the whisked egg whites into the egg yolks. Sift in the coconut flour and almond flour and fold in until well combined.

Pour the mixture into the pan and spread evenly. Bake in the oven for about 15 minutes. When done, remove from the oven and let cool. Cut into ladyfinger shapes or squares.

Meanwhile, prepare the mascarpone layer. Separate the egg yolks from the egg whites. Whisk the egg whites with a pinch of salt and gradually add half of the powdered erythritol while whisking into stiff peaks. Set aside.

Place the egg yolks into a heat-resistant bowl. Beat the egg yolks with the liquid stevia and the remaining erythritol until pale and creamy. Place the bowl on top of a saucepan with simmering water. Cook for about 10 minutes, stirring constantly. Tempering the egg yolks will help keep the mascarpone layer creamy and firm.

Remove from the heat and continue stirring to cool. Fold in the mascarpone cheese. Using a large spoon, slowly fold in some of the whisked egg whites and then the remaining egg whites.

Prepare the coffee liquid. Combine the coffee with the rum or rum extract and the powdered erythritol and liquid stevia. Mix well and then dip each of the ladyfingers into the liquid until soaked but not soggy.

Assemble the trifles by spooning some of the mascarpone mixture into a bowl. Sprinkle with some cacao powder and then add 1 or 2 soaked ladyfingers. Top with another layer of mascarpone, cacao powder, and ladyfingers. Finally, top with more mascarpone and cacao powder.

Chill in the fridge for at least a few hours or overnight. Cover each trifle with plastic wrap to prevent the top from drying out.

TIP

Is alcohol keto-friendly? Clear spirits, such as vodka, whiskey, and tequila are zero-carb, and a glass of dry wine is considered low-carb. However, your body can't store alcohol as fat: it has to metabolize it, and the result is that your body will burn it instead of fat for fuel. That means you shouldn't have a large dinner and drink alcohol at the same time. Also, be aware that ketosis will lower your tolerance for alcohol.

CHAI TEA PANNA COTTA

Your guests will love this lightly spiced, tea-infused dessert.
It's very low in carbs, and it's so simple to make.

 6 SERVINGS | **10 MINS** | **20 MINS** + CHILLING

INGREDIENTS

2 cups (480 ml/16.2 fl oz) almond milk

1½ cups (360 ml/12.2 fl oz) heavy whipping cream or coconut milk

1 tablespoon (7 g/0.3 oz) gelatin powder, preferably grass-fed, or 1 teaspoon agar powder

¼ cup (60 ml/2 fl oz) water

¼ cup (40 g/1.4 oz) erythritol or Swerve, powdered

10 to 15 drops stevia

Chai Tea Spices
1 vanilla bean

2 cinnamon sticks

4 each whole cloves, black peppercorns

8 cardamom pods, crushed

1 teaspoon each fennel seeds, and ground ginger
(or 1 tablespoon ginger)

¼ teaspoon each allspice, nutmeg and salt

2 to 3 tablespoons (4 to 6 g/ 0.1 to 0.2 oz) loose black tea

Cut the vanilla bean lengthwise and scrape the seeds into a saucepan using a sharp knife. Add the rest of the spices, salt, and tea, then the almond milk and cream: this is the chai tea concentrate.

Bring to a boil over a low heat and simmer for about 10 minutes. Take it off the heat and cover with a lid. Let the mixture infuse for 20 minutes. Pour the cream through a fine mesh sieve or cheesecloth into another saucepan. Discard the spices.

Sprinkle the gelatin into the water and mix until well combined. Add the erythritol and liquid stevia to the cream-and-chai mixture and slowly bring to a boil. Remove from the heat, add the bloomed gelatin, and whisk until completely dissolved and smooth.

Pour the chai cream into six small glasses and place in the fridge to set for at least 3 hours or overnight. Cover each glass with plastic wrap to prevent the top from drying out. When ready to serve, sprinkle with ground nutmeg or cinnamon.

NUTRITION FACTS PER SERVING

Total carbs: 3.5 g **Protein:** 2.6 g **Macronutrient ratio:**
Fiber: 0.9 g **Fat:** 23.8 g Calories from carbs (4%), protein (5%), fat
Net carbs: 2.6 g **Energy:** 239 kcal (91%)

WARMING BERRY POT

This is a low-carb version of a crustless berry cheesecake, and it's a major crowd-pleaser. Make it in advance and keep in the fridge.

 6 SERVINGS | **5 MINS** | **25 MINS**

INGREDIENTS

2 large eggs

8.8 ounces (250 g) cream cheese

½ cup (115 g/4 oz) sour cream

¼ cup (60 ml/2 fl oz) heavy whipping cream or coconut milk

2 tablespoons (20 g/0.7 oz) erythritol or Swerve, powdered

10 to 15 drops stevia

1 tablespoon (15 ml/0.5 fl oz) freshly squeezed lemon juice

1 vanilla bean or 1 teaspoon unsweetened vanilla extract

2 cups (300 g/10.6 oz) fresh or frozen berries (raspberries, strawberries, blackberries and blueberries)

NUTRITION FACTS PER SERVING

Total carbs: 7.7 g

Fiber: 1.5 g

Net carbs: 6.2 g

Protein: 6.1 g

Fat: 20.9 g

Energy: 218 kcal

Macronutrient ratio:
Calories from carbs (10%), protein (10%), fat (80%)

Preheat the oven to 300°F (150°C, or gas mark 2). Wash the berries and pat dry. Whisk together the eggs, cream cheese, sour cream, heavy whipping cream, powdered erythritol, liquid stevia, lemon juice, and vanilla. Mix in the berries. Pour into a casserole dish or 6 individual ramekins, and cook for about 20 minutes or until the top is caramelized. Eat warm or let it cool and store in the fridge.

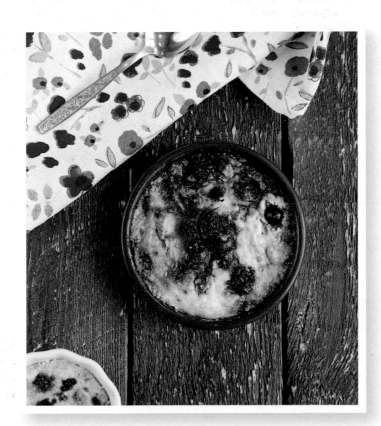

INDEX

About the Author

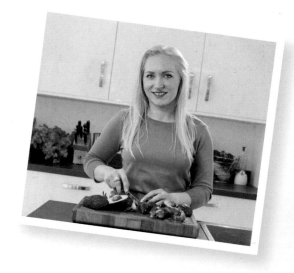

Martina Slajerova is a health and food blogger living in the United Kingdom. She holds a degree in economics and worked in auditing, but has always been passionate about nutrition and healthy living. Martina loves food, science, photography, and creating new recipes. She is a firm believer in low-carb living and regular exercise. As a science geek, she bases her views on valid research and has firsthand experience of what it means to be on a low-carb diet. Both are reflected on her blog, in her KetoDiet apps, and this book.

The KetoDiet is an ongoing project she started with her partner in 2012 and includes *The KetoDiet Cookbook* and the KetoDiet apps for the iPad and iPhone (www.ketodietapp.com). When creating recipes, she doesn't focus on just the carb content: You won't find any processed foods, unhealthy vegetable oils, or artificial sweeteners in her recipes.

This book and the KetoDiet apps are for people who follow a healthy low-carb lifestyle. Martina's mission is to help you reach your goals, whether it's your dream weight or simply eating healthy food. You can find even more low-carb recipes, diet plans, and information about the keto diet on her blog: www.ketodietapp.com/blog.